Leadership in Retrospect: From the Stretcher-Side to the Boardroom

by Antoinette Weathers, MSN, RN, CEN-R

with Christopher Card, Ph.D.

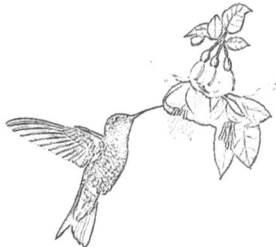

Dedication

Nurses are the best part of the worst day in many people's lives. Moreover, they never lose sight that what they consider routine is often life-changing for patients and their loved ones. Cheryl, a former nursing director, recounted a comment from a family member that sums it up best: "Nurses are angels without wings, but they sure can fly!"

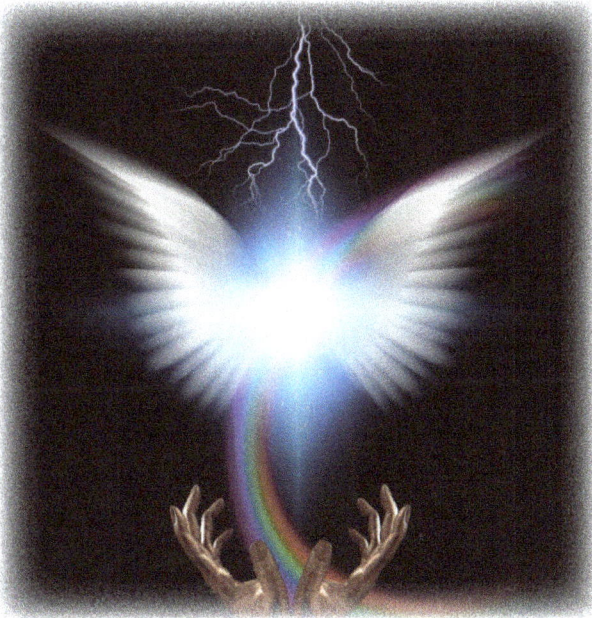

To all of the courageous frontline nurses who battled Covid-19:
Your voice, the touch of your hands, and your presence are the last
things many people experience in this world.
God put you at the stretcher-side for a reason.
For nurses are to our health care system as angels are to Heaven.

Contents

Foreword by Christopher Card, Ph.D.

Antoinette "Stormy" Weathers, or Toni, (as she is known by her friends) is a wealth of information and a goldmine of sincere caring, powerful wisdom, and plain charisma wrapped into a five-foot, one-hundred-pound frame. She writes with her heart wide open and shares her most precious gems of quality leadership and nursing skills in this book—telling all in a conversational, yet very professional manner.

The book is truly a boon to new leaders and those already in administrative positions. It explains the highlights of what to expect and gives powerful examples of real-life scenarios plus tried-and-true theories and practices. My role has been a labor of love alongside Stormy, editing the manuscript and providing little suggestions where I could, as well as coordinating the visual imagery.

This is no ordinary leadership text, nor is it a reminiscing of a past career. Antoinette has a stalwart past with twenty-plus years in management and leadership, having been an Emergency Department Manager and Professional Development Coordinator and in other leadership roles throughout her nursing career. She believes strongly, as I do, in life-long learning, and it shows in her background.

She is a self-made professional who has spent a lifetime working in healthcare while continuing her education. She has completed numerous post graduate courses and maintains the highest standards of professional practice. I am pleased to call her a friend and confidant and continue to learn from her advice and golden guidebook of wisdom.

This book will change your vision of leadership, particularly the Conceptual Framework and model she presents in chapter two, setting the tone in such an eloquent way for all she says in the other sections of this book by presenting the lifestyle that she, herself, leads.

Toni, as a true friend and colleague, utters her own unique words in this tome which will reach beyond the scope of the nursing world and into leadership texts and courses throughout the globe. This book shall remain timely for years to come as it outlines some of the most cutting-edge concepts in leadership in a very accessible and professional manner. The new directions it presents are sure to inspire. Use this book as your blueprint for leadership and management, regardless of your field or direction. Advice, wisdom, theories, and concepts like these are truly educationally life changing.

Preface

To a treasured friend, co-author, scholar, and wordsmith, Chris
Card. We began with a stack of tattered pages from a diary. He
worked long and hard to turn the notes into a comprehensible
work and deserves much credit. If anything within these pages is
wrong, the fault is mine. If, however, the content is decipherable,
then Chris is foremost the one who deserves the credit.

- "Stormy"

Acknowledgements

Writing a book is harder than we thought and more rewarding than we ever imagined.
It would not have come to fruition without the love and support of family and friends.
Chris and I want to give our heartfelt thanks to:

Robyn and Paul

Extra special thanks to our spouses Robyn Card and Paul Weathers for being there for us, tirelessly, through this special journey and assisting behind the scenes with support and encouragement.

The Slackers: Steve and Renae Adrian

For their generous hospitality in a beautiful home where friends make memories and always find just the right mix of solitude and laughter.
Smith Mountain Lake is a writer's paradise.

Our beta reader: Linda Whitt, BSN, RN, CEN-R

Admired deeply for her qualities and considered an expert by her colleagues in the medical and nursing professions.

Our diligent editor, award-winning author, publisher, and friend: Dawn Brotherton.

The world is a better place when people take time to mentor others. Like a great teacher, Dawn stretched us beyond our comfort zones, transforming writers into authors.

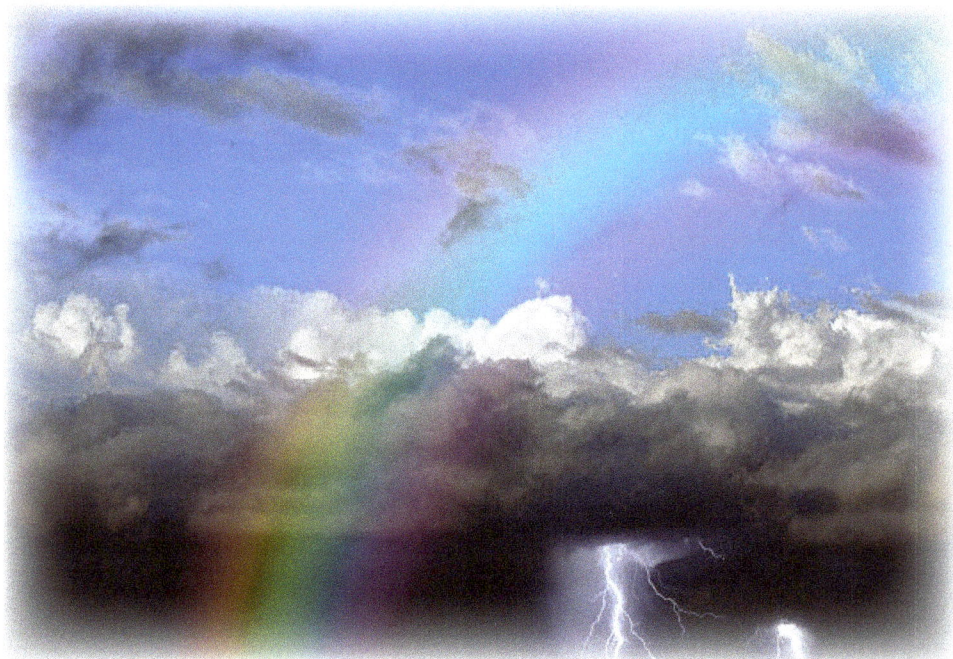

Introduction

Good judgment comes from experience, and experience—well, that comes from poor judgment. Anon.

- Anonymous

Leadership in Retrospect: From the Stretcher-Side to the Boardroom casts light upon fundamental best practices and pearls of wisdom acquired during a healthcare career spanning over forty years. I have a desire to encourage and support future leaders in healthcare by paying lessons forward. The professional development of others is a personal passion and the primary purpose of this book. In this way, knowledge becomes a gift, creating a legacy and ongoing cycle for mentoring.

I don't recommend dwelling upon the past any more than looking in the rearview mirror while driving forward, but we should be mindful of what is behind us as well as what is lurking in our blind spots. A retrospective review can be helpful *if* we reflect to learn, not to dwell. After all, there is no such thing as failure, only mistakes that inform us how to become better. Unfortunately, people who fail to talk, write, or think about mistakes are destined to repeat them.

The school of hard knocks provided me with ample oppor-tunities to learn and grow. I've endured turbulent times veiled by dark, foreboding clouds. At times, lightning would strike with an illuminating lesson and brighten the stormy weather. Sometimes I was blessed with a brilliant rainbow after a storm and looked over the rainbow to discover precious gold nuggets of wisdom on the other side. I hope you unearth a few gold nuggets for yourself in the shelter of this book. My grandfather Richard once said, "When you find something of value, the first thing you should do is go out and share it." He was right.

The lessons I recount in these pages can help you successfully navigate the nursing profession, whether you are at the bedside, stretcher-side, or in a boardroom. You will be able to apply much of the information to your daily work tomorrow. The format is concise, with a laser focus on ideas in anecdotes, examples, and bullet points. Highlight it. Mark it up and document personal experiences, ideas, observations, and lessons. Make this book a well-thumbed reference as you chronicle your nursing journey.

Along the way, take time to notice the rainbows and silver-linings in the clouds. Celebrate successes and learn from them as well. We often hear about learning from mistakes, but also learn from your achievements. Then, write your story and pass it on. I pray you will always be safe and have an angel on your shoulder wherever your journey takes you.

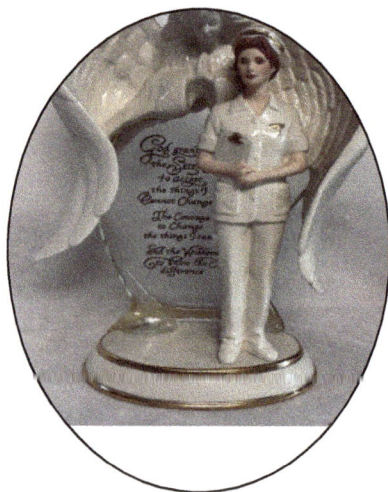

Angel on Your Shoulder

Part One

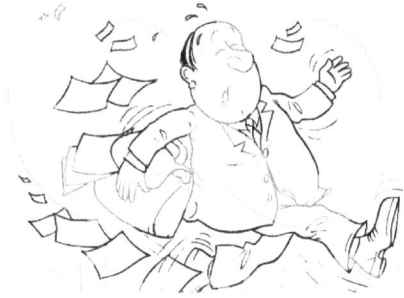

Chapter One:
The Accidental Manager: Is This You?

Most of what you read about leadership sounds like common sense and appears easy to accomplish, but at least in my experience (if not yours), it's not common practice. Sometimes leadership capabilities, such as motivating others, team building, and conflict resolution, are referred to as soft skills. That has always baffled me because management and leadership are very challenging! Just look around your organization. How many good leaders can you identify? There are very few people who can lead effectively if your organization is like most. I believe people are often unprepared as they begin their first assignments managing others. To complicate matters further, the people they are managing may have been their peers.

In a 2019 benchmark survey of the emergency, trauma, and transport nursing workforce, 38.5% of respondents cited a need for leadership/management training and explicitly reported a need for efficient, competent leaders (Schumaker et al., 2019). Perhaps this is because many people in management positions are what I refer to as *accidental managers*; they enter into their roles in a haphazard and unplanned manner. Worse, once promoted, people don't always receive the support, training, and professional development needed to be successful.

The Peter Principle, first articulated by Laurence Peter, also adds to the problem of unqualified managers (Wikipedia Contributors, 2019). Typically, we begin our careers working in a specific area or performing particular functions in the organization. We become very proficient in our roles. Our technical skills, expertise, and performance create enough momentum that we are noticed and then promoted just above the competence level where we function best.

I feel comfortable stating this opinion because I was once an accidental manager and a byproduct of the Peter Principle. I stumbled into management. One day I was in an education role, then the next day, I was the nurse manager. The knowledge, skills, and abilities (KSAs) I possessed as an educator provided credibility in the high-tech world of healthcare, but I lacked the wisdom and experience for competence in management and leadership roles. Many mistake KSAs for wisdom. They are not the same things.

I quickly learned that clinical subject matter expertise (knowledge) does not make one wise. It's the application of knowledge, skills, and abilities to everyday life that constitutes wisdom. What is the value and practicality of something if you know it but don't know how to use it? I needed to polish skills such as delegation and communication, giving feedback, and having difficult conversations—the so-called soft skills. Having strong technical knowledge was not enough. Success in the new role required adaptability, agility, and motivation to reinvent my former self.

The lesson here is being good at one job does not guarantee one will easily transition and do well in another position. Organizations would be wise to reward based on performance and promote based on competencies required for the job. Promotions should be reserved for those who clearly can handle the next career step, not just for superior performance at the current level. Organizations must develop people, design succession planning strategies, and offer mentoring programs for bench strength. Leadership is a learned behavior. By proactively managing talent, the organization will have people in the pipeline ready to step up to the next level of responsibility.

Be prepared for the next opportunity! All of us have weaknesses. The strategy is to determine which ones can be improved, then get to work on those. Don't let your leadership style develop accidentally.

Reflection

1. How did you get to be in the position you're in? Are you an *accidental manager?*

2. Identify a minimum of two personal coaching needs. For example, are you comfortable with engaging in crucial conversations? Have you mastered the art and skill of public speaking?

3. Create a list of three prospective mentors. Reflect upon their attributes as you read the following sections.

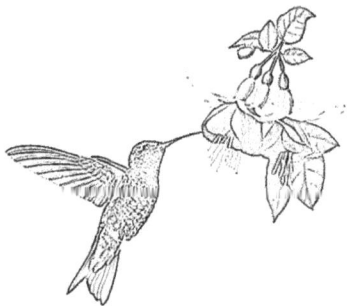

Chapter Two:
A Conceptual Framework:
Leadership Domains of Success

A group of managers attended a leadership conference. The facilitator opened the session with a simple group exercise. Everyone was given a blank sheet of paper with instructions to take five minutes and list what needed to be changed in their organization. Here's what some of the participants wrote:

"The CEO needs to get a backbone!"

"We need more staff and resources."

"Replace the outdated office furniture."

"We have too many meetings."

"My co-workers lack accountability."

Other responses were similar. Yet, no one in the audience wrote, "I need to change."

Always look to yourself first. As leaders, we must role model the language of accountability. Ask the right questions. Begin inquiries with what and how, not why, when, or who. For example, "What can I do to develop myself?" and "How can I help?" Focus on "I," not them.

What's the Secret Sauce for Survival and Success?

I once read many newly placed executives fail within their first eighteen months. This fact resonated with me since I worked as a staff nurse in an emergency department notorious for rapid turnover among managers and directors. Unfortunately, there is no holy grail of leadership.

So, what are the drivers of achievement? How does one not only survive but also thrive and find joy throughout the journey? This section introduces a conceptual model for leadership survival and success in the twenty-first century, focusing on the three big Cs: Collaboration, Connections, and Communication, plus, of paramount importance: You!

I can almost hear the sighs. "Not a model!"

But don't shy away. The framework is offered for visual learners (like me) to help organize our thinking and envision how complex relationships work together. Self-refinement is at the apex.

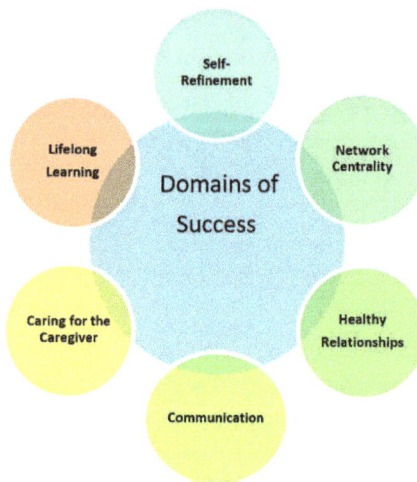

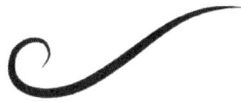

Domain One: Self-Refinement

Watch your thoughts, they become words;
Watch your words, they become actions;
Watch your actions, they become habits;
Watch your habits, they become character;
Watch your character, for it becomes your destiny.

(Goodreads, 2021, Frank Outlaw section)

Character is defined by Merriam-Webster (1991) as moral excellence, and it is a trait often attributed to leaders. As individuals, it's essential to recognize the value of character and do what is needed to uphold personal and organizational values.

Core values are our fundamental beliefs or guiding principles that inform our decisions and dictate our behavior. Take a few moments to reflect upon your core values before continuing. What are your organization's core values, and are they congruent with your personal ones?

It's likely we share many of the same tenets.

Treating everyone with respect and dignity. A simple practice to adopt is to remember the names of people as well as something good about them, if possible. This includes becoming acquainted with the receptionists, environmental service and maintenance workforce, people who keep the software securely updated, deliver food trays, and others with whom you interact on a routine basis.

Being kind. Clothe yourself in compassion. Perform *Acts of Kindness* (Sandel, 2021*).* Self-compassion—simply giving the same kindness to ourselves that we give to others—is equally important.

Accepting people for who they are and peering beyond unfavorable qualities to see the good. Admittedly, I was not always forgiving of others. Amy, an insightful boss, helped me realize I had a "burn them at the stake" mentality. Her words, not mine. Please don't judge me too harshly; I've already done that for you. Besides, my past sins carry their own punishments. A merciless, unforgiving temperament did not serve me well. Living life every day as if everything had to be perfect only made those around me miserable. Fortunately, I've learned we must be tolerant of mistakes. Don't cling to a need for perfection in yourself or in others. It will drive people away. Perfection is attained only in the most fleeting of moments, and if you spend your life failing to attain it over and over again, you are going to end up with a life full of anguish and disappointment. Besides, have you noticed the only people who don't make mistakes are those who never do anything?

Keeping commitments and promises builds trust. It's one thing to talk about noble intentions and make pledges, but action is the best measure of fidelity. It can be challenging to keep track of promises you've made as new ones eclipse your time and attention. Find a simple method to track promises. If an adjustment becomes necessary in fulfilling a commitment, then communicate the modification and make a recommitment.

Steadfastly giving your best effort, even when you don't want to. Steadfastly giving your best effort means consistently working toward what is important to you. No success is immediate, and no collapse is sudden. Both outcomes are the result of the momentum accrued through repetitive daily actions. Julius Erving, a former basketball superstar, once said, "Being a professional is doing things you love to do, (even) on the days you don't feel like doing them" (Pink, 2009, p. 123). Put forth your best every day, and over time, your efforts yield a monumental positive impact.

Consistently taking a stand for what is right. Never backstab. It's especially important to avoid idle gossip and always be loyal to those who are not present. In this way, you build the trust and respect of those present. An experienced trauma nurse knows ABCDE stands for Airway, Breathing, Circulation, Disability, Expose, and Environment (though not always in that sequence). However, to those who lack integrity, ABCDE can also stand for Accuse, Belittle, Criticize, Demoralize, and Expunge.

Remember, we judge ourselves based on our intentions, but others judge us based on our behavior. Therefore, we must exercise morality and employ congruency between our best intentions and our actions. Good leaders model a positive, optimistic attitude.

Attitude is the mindset or viewpoint that reflects our feelings toward the environment and other people. Simply put, it is our paradigm of the world, and it's impacted by the circumstances we encounter. More importantly, however, attitude affects our response or how we react to those situations. A stimulus is under someone else's control or no one's power (as in a natural disaster), but your reaction is always under your command. You control how you respond to things. It's even possible to alter our physiology and lives by altering our attitudes. Don't give the freedom and power of a healthy perspective away! The following situation illustrates this point.

One day a nurse entered my office furious and visibly upset after a dispute with one of her coworkers. We discussed the incident, and then I remarked, "You are response-able."

She was stunned because she mistakenly assumed I said, "You are responsible," instead of correctly hearing, "You are response-able."

I clarified that we determine and control our responses. There is always a gap between a stimulus and our reaction to it. I've never regretted practicing self-regulation by keeping a filter on impulses and emotions in check, allowing silence, and pausing before responding to a stimulus. It's during this brief pause that I ask, "Is what I'm about to do a reflection of who I am and who I want to be?" Just STOP.

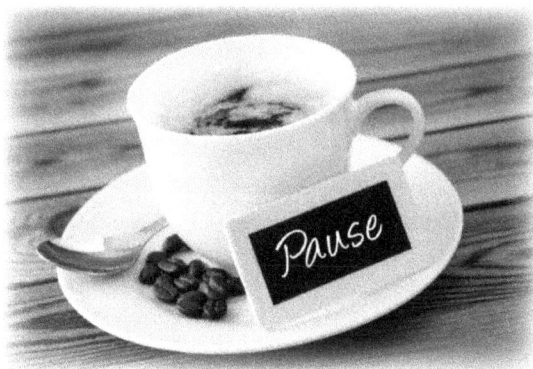

Stop and pause for a cause.

Take a deep breath.

Observe what you are doing.

Proceed.

I had regrets when I reacted too quickly with words and actions. It's often been those times I wanted to take things back, but it was too late.

Our thoughts in this momentary pause will power us to react in an appropriate way. We supply internal dialogue and meaning to the event. We are the ones feeding the ideas—whether the self-talk is positive or negative. We can make a conscious choice to choose an optimistic or pessimistic perspective.

Of course, a positive paradigm doesn't imply we wear blinders to minimize or ignore unwanted incidents and poor behaviors. Adverse incidents are still explored, just not with gut-wrenching blame and anger. Instead, we explore events with curiosity, an inquisitive mindset, and a different lens. You can transform the environment, or it will transform you.

In the extreme, individuals who faced great suffering and adversity have shared their remarkable stories. Notably, Viktor E. Frankl, psychiatrist and Holocaust survivor reminds us:

We who lived in concentration camps can remember the men who walked through the huts comforting others, giving away their last piece of bread. They may have been few in number, but they offer sufficient proof that everything can be taken from a man but one thing: the last of the human freedoms—to choose one's attitude in any given set of circumstances, to choose one's own way. (A-Z Quotes, n.d., Victor E. Frankl quote)

Victor Frankl was unable to control his suffering and adversity, but he did control how he responded. As a result, he maintained a strong mindset, which was a powerful force that allowed him to overcome hardship and survive.

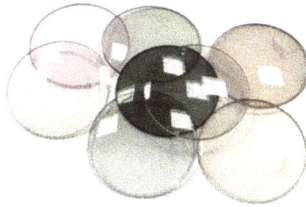

Using the Proper Lens of Vision

Fortunately, most of us will never endure such hardship, but we encounter challenges, fears, and annoyances every day. The person you are and your collective experiences color how you see the world and everything in it. It is your lens.

One way to reframe your attitude is by looking at a situation with a reverse lens. In other words, put yourself in the opposite position or from the other person's perspective. In the case described above, the reverse lens allowed the nurse to understand the situation and build a level of empathy for the other person's point of view. The process may have been a little painful, but she also gained self-awareness of her first reaction (to fight or take flight) and the power to control her response.

I recently watched Freaky Friday. This film is an example of what I refer to as edutainment (educational constructs conveyed through entertainment). It's a 2003 Disney movie directed by Mark Waters and written by Heather Hach and Leslie Dixon, based on Mary Rodgers's 1972 novel of the same name. The original film features Jamie Lee Curtis and Lindsay Lohan as a mother and daughter, respectively, whose bodies are magically switched. Each is forced to walk in the other's shoes for one "Freaky Friday." Through this experience, they gain an appreciation of the difficulties the other faces and begin to experience life through the lens of one another. Essentially, they developed empathy for each other.

Empathy is being able to understand and acknowledge another person's situation, feelings, and motives. The key word in this definition is *feelings*. When you're empathizing with another person, you're trying to understand what it feels like to be in that person's situation.

Don't confuse empathy with sympathy. The terms are similar but do not share the same meaning. Both empathy and sympathy come from a good place—our hearts. The primary difference is how they make the one who is hurting feel. Sympathy is feeling pity for another's loss or misfortune. It can make a grieving person feel more isolated and may even produce an unbalanced power dynamic. On the other hand, empathy is understanding what another person is feeling. You and the other person are on an equal platform because you may have experienced the same situation yourself or you can at least imagine being in the same circumstances.

When an employee or colleague comes to you with an issue or problem, it's so easy to jump right into problem-solving mode. My husband tends to leap right into "fix-it" mode when I'm only expressing a viewpoint and seeking validation. He quickly begins to propose solutions, and that irritates me further because I don't feel heard and understood.

When you're trying to understand someone's feelings, first observe what they say or how they are acting. Are they overwhelmed or frustrated? Then, acknowledge that they're in a really tough bind, or they have a lot on their plate. It's helpful to use open-ended phrases such as, "Help me to understand why you . . ." or "Can you tell me more about . . . because I want to understand what you are thinking and feeling."

When we are attuned to the feelings of others and recognize their concerns, we're more successful in our relationships. As a manager, you can also use the reverse lens approach to help your team members develop a better understanding of each other. This insight into another's perspective develops team cohesiveness.

Further, consider empathy in the context of customer service. Displaying empathy must come before problem-solving—order matters. Remember the adage that no one cares how much you know until they know how much you care.

Reframing with a Longer and Wider Lens

Another way to reframe and renew your attitude is to look at the situation with a long lens. Consider the situation in six months or in a year from now. Will it even matter tomorrow? If there are long term implications, then what can you do today to ensure the outcome is successful? This approach allows you to gain perspective on the current situation so you can avoid overreacting.

Still another way to reframe and renew your attitude is to look at the situation with a wide lens. Challenge yourself and ask the question, "How can I grow from this experience or situation?"

Conditions that are very daunting are often opportunities for learning and for personal or professional development. By maintaining a positive attitude and practicing pragmatic optimism, you are better able to turn adversity into an opportunity that fosters success.

Finally, avoid the dreaded Four Ps of Pessimism:

Personal: There's something wrong with me; they don't like me. Why do bad things always happen to me? For example, if someone cancels a date, it must be because a better offer came along. This distorted cognitive reasoning, known as personalization, leads to stress and anxiety.

Instead, practice being mindful of the tendency to blame yourself when things don't go as planned. Look outside yourself for more rational explanations. Often it isn't clear why people behave as they do. To take everyone's behavior personally isn't fair to others and not kind to yourself.

Permanent: Things will never get any better.

Try to look through the long lens. It's unlikely that the situation will last forever. Setbacks are usually temporary. Feelings dampen with the tincture of time.

Pervasiveness: Global mindset—the problem is affecting my personal life, professional life, relationships, my home, my whole life!

Look through the wide lens. Remember, problems often affect only one area and are not a colossal indication that something is wrong with the totality of your universe.

Poor Perspective: We often exhaust ourselves with worry about trifling matters. Nurses know *shiFt* happens. We ruin our favorite uniform with blood stains (and other unmentionable things). The cafeteria customer in line ahead of us can't decide what to order, and we only have a thirty-minute break. The next shift is late, and now we can't leave work on time.

Don't waste time and energy worrying about insignificant things. If something doesn't matter one year from now, then don't let it squander another minute from your life. Accept what you cannot control. You will save energy by choosing to let go of trivial things out of your control.

Refining yourself begins with self-awareness and acceptance. Each person has a unique combination of strengths. If we identify and focus on our top strengths, it will have a lasting effect on our overall well-being.

A key to forming meaningful human relationships is the capacity to appreciate others' strengths. No one expects leaders to be experts in everything, but we do need to know who is skilled and knowledgeable in certain areas and where we can find resources. Be self-aware of personal weaknesses and find others to fill in these gaps.

What's your superpower? If you are a nurse, then I believe you are a star. We are all stars; some of us just need polishing to sparkle and shine like superstars. Then we can make the world a brighter and better place.

Reflection

1. The most important investment you can make is in yourself. What can you do today to become a better version of yourself?

2. What are your top character strengths? List several, such as optimism, gratitude, perseverance, or others.

3. What character fortes do you appreciate in others?

4. What talents can you master to maximize your potential?

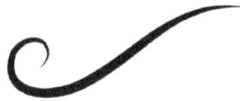

Domain Two: Network Centrality

Take an interest in others before they take an interest in you.

(Maxwell, 2007, p.45)

Do you know secret societies exist in many organizations? They do. There is also a method to uncover and identify the exclusive members, those few who are powerful. However, before continuing, we must define power and differentiate between two distinct forms.

According to Daft (2016), power is the capacity of a person or group to influence others to achieve desired outcomes. Legitimate power is the authority vested by the organizational position and by reporting relationships, not necessarily because of the leader's characteristics. Legitimate power flows down a vertical hierarchy and along the chain of command. Someone can have a title that gives them much authority yet, in reality, possess little real power and not be influential.

Personal or referent power stems from credibility; people believe in and respect leaders with referent power. Informal leaders often derive power from a repertoire of knowledge, skills, and abilities. We follow these true leaders not because we must, but because we want to. Additionally, these successful powerholders may also possess political acumen and weave intricate social webs.

Here is the big reveal. Informal powerholders are members of the secret society who hold substantial shares of social capital. Their names are not always portrayed on an organizational chart. Yet, they are central figures in the organization with access to people and information channels critical for the company's success. This network centrality culminates in personal power and the ability to wield influence at horizontal and vertical levels in the organization. Members of the secret society are the organization's change champions and often act as brokers connecting different groups.

A technique to discover who these influencers are is social network analysis or SNA (Pollack & Matous, 2019). It's beyond the scope of this work to provide a detailed academic explanation of SNA. In brevity, social network analysis uses data, statistics, and other techniques to uncover work relationships, power structure, and leadership potential. Using SNA, we can find who people turn to for answers and where much of the work is accomplished. This alone can prove priceless to an organization.

For example, this analysis can determine who the real experts are so their knowledge can be shared and stored before separation or retirement.

Cultivating Network Centrality

How does one develop network centrality? The concept of network centrality entails so much more than physical space, but simple location can be a crucial factor if it increases your visibility and access to people.

Appearance, such as office decor, is also a consideration, especially in creating good first impressions. This may seem trivial, but it was once a personal albatross of mine. My office was a cramped, cinderblock, broom closet adjacent to a noisome bathroom on a corridor used for storage. The space reminded me of the tiny closet at the foot of the stairs in J. K. Rowling's *Harry Potter and the Sorcerer's Stone*.

Ironically, my office was also the place where new hires reported for on-boarding! It's a rhetorical question, but is there anyone who cannot agree this was thoughtless and shortsighted? (Please pardon the digression, but there is great therapeutic value in the catharsis that comes with lancing emotional boils.)

Aside from location, network centrality is also fostered by going the extra mile, taking on projects, developing expertise, and acquiring knowledge vitally important to the company. Yet don't be myopic by looking only within your organization because you will miss significant trends.

Network in multiple venues:

- Build alliances within the community and join professional organizations.
- Participate in conferences at regional and national levels.
- Contribute to evidence-based, intellectual dialogue, such as in professional blogs and digests. If you ever have an opportunity to present a topic, embrace it and, if possible, share the materials far and wide. Make sure to put as much polish on the presentation as you can. Members of our profession don't have to keep reinventing the wheel when we take the time to share with others.
- Keep business cards on you at all times and try to accumulate cards from people in your field, then follow up with those people and keep the connections alive.
- Finally, we must also act politically in the workplace at times. In the past, I thought of office politics with negative connotations, such as self-serving behavior. On the contrary, political action is sometimes required to build consensus around issues, especially when uncertainty is high, and there is discord over priorities. Politically influential leaders know who the members of the secret society are and understand influence flows mostly from relationships, not job titles. To act politically, one must be aware of the stakeholders' interests. Whose support is needed if we want to implement a change or have our point of view prevail? What is the most effective way to

gain support? Who are the key players loyal to? What might make it easy (or difficult, as the case may be) to gain their acceptance and approval?

A Final Note on Power

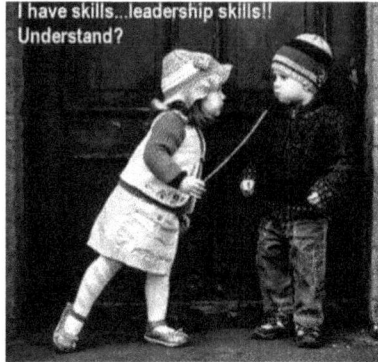

As you develop network centrality, remember to use your newly acquired power wisely. Power should not be flaunted or abused in a coercive fashion. People don't like power hounds.

I had an amateurish boss who resorted to coercion and creating a toxic environment of fear. Fortunately, I had options and separated when she allocated an impossible workload as a fait accompli, leaving no room for discussion.

People want respect and autonomy, and anyone who tries to lead through intimidation and fear will only be successful for a short period of time. Publicizing one's power is not necessary. People already know who has power.

Power works its magic best when it's covert. To draw attention to power is to lose it. Like President Theodore Roosevelt's well-known motto regarding foreign policy, "Speak softly, and carry a big stick; you will go far" (Wikipedia Contributors, 2019a).

Having power and carrying a big stick is a definite bonus. You never know when you are going to need to tap into power stores to accomplish critical initiatives. However, don't use it if you don't need to.

Reflection

1. Do people in your organization have power based primarily on their position in the hierarchy or based on other factors, such as their knowledge, skills, and abilities?

2. Can you identify any key powerholders in your organization who are not on the organizational chart? Are you one of them?

3. Do you get along with most everyone? Certainly, there are a few difficult people, but in general, can you co-exist peacefully with most people?

4. Are you approachable and available to those around you? Do people naturally come to you and seek you out about interests, problems, joys, or just passing the time?

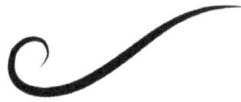

Domain Three: Healthy Relationships

Who you are is who you attract—grow accordingly.

(Maxwell, 2007, p. 203)

The next sphere, contiguous to and intricately related to Network Centrality, is Healthy Relationships. To develop network centrality, many people will need to know who you are and like you. People follow relationships, not titles. Much of the work we do as leaders is accomplished through relationships.

It was often difficult for me to slow down enough to foster meaningful relationships in the past. I even considered water-fountain chit chat or casual conversations a waste of time and detrimental to my productivity. That's regrettable because people, not agendas, are the most significant asset in our lives and to our organizations.

Once we appreciate the tremendous power of relationships and begin to support each other, many of our problems will already be solved (de Vries, 2011). Yet, similar to a successful marriage, one must cultivate and nurture relationships before harvesting the benefits.

We must also inoculate our relationships against real and imagined threats. Resentment, envy, mistrust, and other toxins are destructive and potentially deadly, even when spread in small doses. Strive to spread positive influence, not influenza!

I'll never forget how one person's animosity and distrust went viral and eventually destroyed a Sexual Assault Nurse Examiner (SANE) team. This individual misconstrued even seemingly innocuous gestures as intentional and offensive insults. As a case in point,

38

I gave all team members wallet-sized plastic cards with tipping rate charts for quick, easy reference during business dinners and travel. You've probably seen these laminated guides on how much currency to tip for services.

This individual responded to the gesture with contempt, claiming I was insulting her math skills. She could have spared everyone the conflict by merely assuming good intentions. It's exhausting to work at cross purposes because it requires so much more energy and effort.

Yet, if you are a nurse, then you are undoubtedly familiar with the paradox of how members of the most trusted profession in the world can be so incredibly brutal to their own. You've even probably heard the expression we "eat our young."

Here is another secret: We also "eat our old." Workplace bullying among nurses is an occupational hazard. No discussion on relationships in nursing would be complete without mentioning this phenomenon of normalized social deviance, so there it is. Now, let's do something about it.

As leaders, we can end this cycle of violence by creating a culture where positive human dynamics are as essential to one's success as factors related to technical skills. If you see bullying, then don't avoid or ignore it. We lower the bar when we go silent. Even worse, we become accomplices when we don't speak up. Trust with individual accountability, perseverance, skilled communication, and constructive conflict resolution are fundamental elements in a healthy, world-class team.

Similarly, keep in mind that what is best for one person is typically best for the other team member(s). If one person succeeds, then everyone benefits. We can also take lessons from other professional groups.

If you want to experience a real-world example of teams and relationships, go to a concert hall and observe musicians in a symphony orchestra. A masterful performance requires collaboration, discipline, complementarity of talent, and role clarity, such as identifying each section's leader or principal.

During rehearsals, great performers are attentive to constructive feedback. They want to be at their best, and therefore, they cultivate relationships in a way that other professionals are comfortable approaching them to point out blind spots. These blind spots are personal shortcomings and flaws of which an individual is unaware (not able to perceive in oneself) but are noticeably apparent and well-known to others.

By accepting feedback from others, the musicians head off mistakes that may negatively impact live performances. The outcome is perfect harmony.

One additional point is blind spots become even more pronounced as we move higher in power and prestige. We need to be aware of this and remember, even as principal players, there is much we have not yet mastered. There's always room to improve, and we can learn from one another.

Purposeful Rounding Up and Down and All Around

Although it does take effort to build healthy relationships, there are tools and tips to make our jobs easier and more effective. One way to foster relationships in the workplace is to be curious about people and maintain a sense of wonder.

Manage by walking around. Good leaders don't just sit in their office and wait for someone to knock on the door with a problem. They get out and talk to people in the organization. They make observations and ask questions to learn more about what their employees do and to understand their challenges. For example, have you ever sat in the unit secretary's chair at a nurses' station? If not, try doing it for an hour to truly appreciate the challenges of the unit secretary position. It is a humbling experience.

Incidentally, a bonus to managing by walking around is that it decreases the volume of emails. If you regularly round, then others will not have the need to email you as often. I've always found it's easier to talk things over during a "curbside" conversation or consult than in email dialogues. As you round, do not forget that your relationships up the chain are just as meaningful as your relationships with the people you supervise.

Take time to sit down and talk with people about their interests and families (including the four-legged household members). Show a genuine interest in getting to know your employees. You should not pry into their personal lives; however, if an employee or coworker shares personal details, you should respond as any benevolent human being would. If a spouse has been ill, then express compassion. If someone shares that a son or daughter is leaving for college, show interest in how they settle in. Exhibiting personal interest conveys a sense of caring that is very important to individuals. However, the concern cannot be fake, and this is not a "one and done" task to be checked off on a long list of to-dos.

"Rounding Logs" and "Favorite's Lists" are two practical tools, especially if you have several team members. A rounding log can be a simple spreadsheet or document as depicted in the figure below or as complex as a specialized software program designed for mobile devices.

Date	Employee	Rounding Note with Details	Follow-Up
28 Aug	Allison Stehley	Son (John) left for college today. Football scholarship to Notre Dame.	3 Sept. Team members created and signed a Notre Dame banner for display at Allison's workstation. 15 Sept. During rounding, manager asked about how John is settling in at N.D.

Figure: Format of a simple Rounding Log

I worked with a director who preferred to use traditional index cards. Each day he would check the daily staffing schedule to determine who was working, then he reviewed notecards on these employees before rounding. He also utilized the cards to personalize Christmas greetings and to note significant events, such as employment anniversaries and birthdays. The important point is that people feel more valued and respected when you show you genuinely care and appreciate their unique contributions.

After all, everyone needs to know their job is worthwhile and to feel appreciated by a person in authority. Help employees understand why their jobs matter. Connect the dots between their contributions at work and the positive impact on other people.

When talented employees leave, they take much of the organization's historical knowledge and skills with them. Recruiting, hiring, and training a new employee costs money and takes time. One of the best ways to "close the back door" and retain talent within an organization is through showing appreciation, genuine caring, belongingness, and inclusion. Create an inclusive environment; you don't want employees who feel like they are outsiders, invisible, and anonymous. That spells disaster! Showing gratitude doesn't cost money, and it's something definitely within your control.

Rounding is also an opportunity to let people know their opinions count. Ask questions about tools, equipment, and processes. Find out how they're feeling, what they find frustrating, and what they desire. Ask, "What do you need from me?" It's equally important to close the loop by providing updates on requests. A method to track requests, referred to as "The Stoplight," is described in detail in a subsequent section.

A "Favorites' List" is a fun tool, and most people don't mind completing the questionnaire during the on-boarding process. Create a heading with space for the employee's name and birthday. Customize the form so people can fill in their preferences by categories. Ideas include favorite color, flower/plant, candy, fast food, animal/pet, hobby, author, school/mascot, and sport. Take time to list five more items to include on a "Favorites' List" or explore printable online samples.

1.
2.
3
4.
5.

Keep these forms in the employees' files for easy reference when you want to express appreciation during a difficult shift or celebrate a milestone.

You need to work within legal and organizational restrictions. For example, some items such as gift cards may not be a viable option due to tax reporting or accounting requirements.

A Final Note on Relationships

Don't rely solely on your coworkers and direct reports for all of your social needs. Good relationships with close family members, friends, and others are essential.

We move in the same direction of people within our social circles. Your friends and associates will influence where you go and how you progress on life's journey. That's the reason it's wise to associate with people who are better than yourself. Develop friendships in faith-based organizations, professional groups, civic associations, and special-interest groups, such as book clubs or volunteer agencies.

Most importantly, remember to devote time to your family and close circle of friends. We all have competing priorities.

I'm glad to report I'm making better decisions in the sphere of relationships. I only need an occasional gentle nudge to make the correct choice, and relationships always win in the end!

Reflection

1. List some of your close friends at work. Are they co-workers, subordinates, or superiors?

2. What could be some downsides of close relationships in the workplace?

3. What are some ways to develop cross-functional or matrixed teams within your organization? For example, employees from several departments can work together on projects, such as flu shot clinics or food drives, to make personal connections and break down silos. What are some other interdepartmental activities?

4. What is one social activity a week you can commit to? How will you track your follow-through? The activity can be as simple as having lunch in the cafeteria with a member of your team. As a leader, you set the tone and are an example to your employees through your actions or inactions.

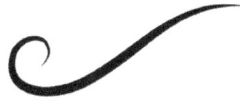

Domain Four: Communication

If speaking is silver, then listening is gold.
(a Turkish proverb as cited in Copeland, 2014, p. 71)

We have two ears, one mouth—<u>for a reason.</u>

Strong communication skills are also a cornerstone of effective leadership. It seems so basic, yet this is one area where most everyone can improve (this author included). I took an introductory course in communications at a community college over forty years ago, but it was decades later before I appreciated the immense value of active listening.

The major problem with communication is most people do not listen with the intent to understand, but rather with the purpose to reply. Leaders need to know how to listen, meaning they should not merely stop talking but be fully present and focused when interacting with others. Control your self-talk and avoid thinking about what you will say in response. Listening at such a deep level requires genuine curiosity, empathy, and a desire to understand.

This entails a capacity to "slip oneself into another's moccasins" and be truly interested in what other people are thinking about.

The first step in becoming a better listener is to have the mindset and desire of wanting to listen. Employees are never an interruption of our work as leaders; they are our work.

View them as stakeholders and contributors in the company rather than paid laborers or staff. A perspective of shared responsibility creates a space in which employees can contribute their feedback on issues that affect the organization. Consideration should be given to the opinions of people who are involved or affected by decisions.

Further, be tactful and respectful of others' opinions even when you disagree. Respect is a continuance issue, meaning if you are not respectful, then the conversation will not continue.

Be mindful of your "hot buttons." When experiencing stress, frustration, and anger, remember you have a choice on how to respond. Here are some helpful strategies for difficult conversations:

- Leave the BMW in the parking lot. No B_ _ _ _ ing, Moaning, or Whining.
- Use silence to buy time.
- Disconnect your feelings from your reactions.
- Use time out when necessary to regain your mental and emotional composure.
- Establish a safety zone, especially if the conversation is sensitive. Do not block yourself into a corner.
- Imagine watching yourself and the situation from a chandelier above. Be objective and think about what you see. What are you doing to help or hinder the situation?

Can You Hear Me Now?

Practice truly listening to people when you go to work tomorrow. As nurses we are problem-solvers, but we need to avoid falling immediately into a "fix-it" mode. Be cognizant of using empathy and active listening skills before offering solutions.

Demonstrate you are fully engaged in the conversation by making good eye contact and voicing attends, as in saying, "Uh huh. I got it. I understand. Keep going." Speakers want encouragement to keep talking. They are looking for affirmation that what they are saying is resonating with the listener. Don't interrupt except as necessary to clarify and confirm. When it's your turn to speak, avoid the use of the word "but." This word is an eraser; it negates what has already been said. For example, "I love you, but . . ." Get the point? Simply start another sentence.

Next, at the risk of stating the obvious, avoid deterrents to active listening. Don't get distracted by looking at your watch or checking your phone or computer. It will appear you are putting the person in front of you in second place. I've been in meetings where I never saw the person's front side, just their rump side!

If you have to use a computer during a meeting, then triangulate the seating arrangement so you are face-to-face with the person, but also able to view the monitor screen. However, remember, it's impossible to multitask!

Finally, it's common knowledge that communication is not all about words. In fact, words are only about 7%. Nonverbal communication accounts for the other 93%. Therefore, it's never enough to say the right thing. You also have to say it the right way. Then, always turn your back before rolling your eyes. (Humor is intended! Don't misinterpret it, especially since all you have is 7% of communication: only my written words.)

Are you rolling your eyes?

I Heard it Through the Grapevine

In a former role as nurse manager, I distributed a weekly newsletter, "The Grapevine." The purpose of the bulletins was to keep everyone up to date while avoiding a dreaded deluge of unread emails. Each topic was limited to three key points. Every issue was composed of a weekly compilation of relevant information including updates on key initiatives, important dates, and employee recognition. In addition to sending the newsletter electronically, I posted copies in the bathroom, on bulletin boards, and in a notebook kept at the nurses' station.

When we communicate, we need to do it often and in many forms. Find the method of communication (phone call, email, text, etc.) that is most appropriate to the situation. Don't rely solely on written forms of communication.

The bottom line is that it's important to keep channels of communication as fluid as possible, even when it's not pleasant. One reason is that bad news early is good news. Further, bad news usually does not get any better with time. However, always be prepared to offer solutions when delivering bad news.

The second reason is we have a need for meaning, so people will fill in the blanks when information is missing or inadequate. It's natural to fill in the facts we don't have—and we rarely, if ever, have all of the facts. This is problematic because we often fill the gaps with unfavorable assumptions. So, what do we add to our memory? We add relative meaning or significance, motive, and judgment (was this a good or bad thing?). The important thing to remember when making sense of situations, events, and conversations is that this is *our* story. It's not necessarily the only valid story. Others will have their interpretations.

To avoid this, it's better to err on the side of over-communicating.

Reflection

1. What type of nonverbal communication do you use most often? What do you see your boss use most often?

2. How can you build rapport with your team?

3. Would daily leadership and unit-based shift huddles be helpful in your organization? Search the internet for examples of huddle agendas that may fit the needs of your department or organization.

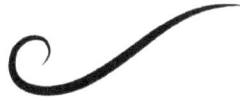

Domain Five: Caring for the Caregiver and Others

Self-care [sic] means giving the world the best of you instead of what is left of you.

(Reed, 2021)

The most important resource we have is ourselves. When you travel on a plane, the flight attendant instructs you to put your oxygen mask on first, before helping others. This is not being selfish. Putting your own mask on first is critical because you cannot help anyone else if your oxygen saturation level plummets, and you lose consciousness. Bluntly speaking, if you die, you cannot assist others.

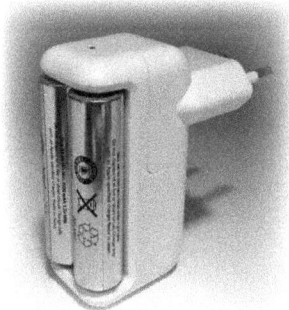

This is also a metaphor for caregivers, including nurses. Caring for others can deplete our energy, strength, and resources. You risk suffering a breakdown when you fail to be attentive to your needs and feelings. Burnout due to excessive demands and depleted reserves will negatively impact mental and physical health, relationships, productivity, and even professional development.

To buffer yourself from burnout, remember: another person's lack of planning is not *your* emergency, and *no* is a complete sentence. Say no (often)!

It is (almost always) appropriate to just say no when you receive a frantic plea to come to work on your one day off or to stay on the job for "just a few more hours" after working a draining twelve-hour shift.

I empathize with managers reading this. I've personally spent countless hours making hundreds of contacts to obtain adequate staff coverage. Incentives, such as premium pay, became the norm for anyone agreeing to work overtime. After a while, even double bonuses were not sufficient to entice people to pick up extra shifts. We eventually reach a tipping point when nothing is as important as having a day off to rest and recuperate.

Nurses, like other workers in high-risk environments, require uninterrupted downtime to refuel and recover from stress. It's a safety and welfare issue for caregivers and their patients.

Here again, we can learn from other professions. Dr. Kevin Gilmartin is a retired police supervisor and psychologist who educated law enforcement on the concept of emotional survival (Grossman & Christensen, 2004). Comparable to police officers, nurses also frequently experience activation of the sympathetic nervous system (SNS) due to the demands and stressors at work. As all nurses know, the SNS keeps us alert and prepared to deal with life and death events. Epinephrine and norepinephrine surge through our bodies, our eyes dilate, digestion slows, heart rate increases, bronchioles relax, glycogen stores are converted to glucose, and blood is shunted to skeletal muscles. These physiological mechanisms keep us going and going and going, even throughout intense twelve-hour shifts.

However, we pay a physiological price for this energizing mechanism. When our long shift ends and we finally go home, the parasympathetic destressing-backlash strikes in the form of exhaustion.

The roller coaster of adrenaline surges followed by backlashes places an incredible toll on our bodies. This is why stress management and recouping energy stores is vital to survival in nursing.

Sleep

You've likely experienced arriving home from work and crashing into a slumber. In meeting our need for sustenance, sleep is as vital to our well-being as water and nutrients. Sleep is not only necessary to rejuvenate, but it also supports the brain's functions for cognition, such as learning and memory.

Grossman and Christensen (2004) portray someone deprived of sleep for twenty-four hours as the psychological and physiologic equivalent of a person in a drunken state. It is common knowledge that sleep deprivation leads to irritability, poor coordination, diminished reflexes, and impaired judgment. Grossman and Christensen cited historical examples of how insufficient sleep has been responsible for major industrial disasters resulting in the loss of many lives and billions of dollars. For instance, Exxon Valdez, Chernobyl, and Three Mile Island had one thing in common: they were all industrial accidents that occurred in the middle of the night involving people with sleep management problems.

For this reason, workers in high-risk industries, such as airline pilots, nuclear plant operators, air traffic controllers, and many others are mandated to get adequate sleep. Yet, healthcare professionals don't always get enough sleep to safely perform their duties.

Clearly, no one wants zombie-like nurses roaming the corridors of hospitals throughout the night. If we were to treat airline pilots and air traffic controllers the way we do our nurses, then planes would be dropping from the sky like hailstones.

Yet, I confess, I've been guilty of asking nurses to work extra shifts and overtime to meet staffing needs without due consideration to the ill effects of sleep deprivation. Before you do the same as a nurse leader, consider the following scenario:

You are a director responsible for an emergency department, and as often the case, you are short on experienced night shift nurses for the upcoming holiday weekend. To compound matters, the charge nurse has just called out sick, and the nurse manager is on vacation.

I come to you from Nurse Agency X and graciously offer to provide nursing coverage for the entire holiday weekend. Great, right? Wait, there are a few drawbacks. I tell you that the available nurses scored below acceptable standards on competency assessments including drug calculations, they are incredibly grumpy, their critical thinking skills are virtually non-existent, and they tend to occasionally doze off. And, by the way, you will need to pay premium wages for the agency nurses. Want them?

The frightening truth is that the Nurse Agency Xers have the same characteristics of our sleep-deprived staff who we've scheduled for excessive overtime! You're not doing the organization—and least of all your patients—any favors by filling in holes on a shift assignment board with the names of tired, warm bodies.

Self-Renewal: The Body, Mind, Heart, and Soul

Stephen Covey (1989) wrote that we are the instruments of our own performance. For this reason, we need to take time regularly to sharpen the saw in all four dimensions: the physical (body), mental (mind), emotional (heart), and spiritual (soul).

The Body

In addition to getting enough sleep, allow time to focus on other physical needs. Do you exercise regularly, eat healthy, schedule wellness activities such as health screenings, and control your weight?

It's been said a formula for longevity is plenty of salad, plenty of bourbon, and plenty of sex. Teach a rabbit to drink, and heck, he may live forever! Alas, unlike the rabbits, we must practice moderation. I keep a quote by Jim Rohn on my refrigerator as a daily reminder. "We must all suffer from one of two pains: the pain of discipline or the pain of regret. What's the difference? Discipline weighs ounces while regret weighs tons" (Taylor, n.d.).

So true. Isn't it interesting that some of life's greatest lessons can be found on magnets stuck to our refrigerator doors?

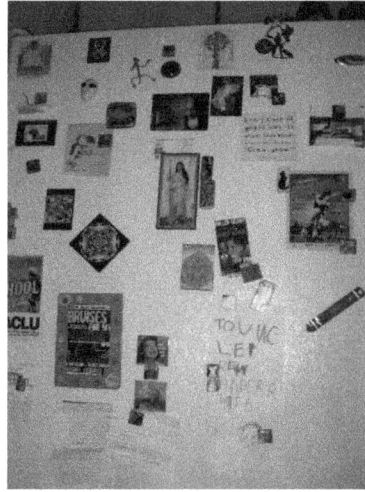

The Mind

Private downtime is not selfish or time squandered. On the contrary, rest and recreation (good old R&R) paradoxically increase our productivity. Yet, the boundaries between work and non-work life are progressively blurred.

There was a time when I worked sixty, sometimes seventy hours, a week. I also suffered a great deal of stress. Admittedly, some of the stress was self-induced, created by my own misperceptions, assumptions, beliefs, and unrealistic expectations. I even slept with my cell phone! What if someone from the hospital needed me in the middle of the night? They usually did call at any and all hours. After all, "What you accept is what you teach" (Cohen, 2007, p.1).

I realize many readers are doing the same because we live in an age of digital deluge, and as nurses, we work 24/7, 365 days a year. The internet and mobile technology allow everyone to work around the clock and from any location. Worse still, we are expected to respond instantly without regard to holidays, weekends, or time of day.

So, how can one survive in an environment of hyperconnectivity? We can use technology wisely, such as limiting alerts and removing screens from the bedroom. Try replacing the smartphone by your bed with a gratitude journal. Then, each night before going to sleep, write down three things you are grateful for—just three good things—and review your journal entries each morning. Ink it, don't just think it!

The demarcation between work and personal life is no longer blurred when you do these simple things. Don't be duped as I once was. There is no such thing as "work-life integration." That is an urban myth and certainly not sustainable in the long run.

Take time for trips. I've always enjoyed air travel. It's interesting to watch people while waiting in airports. Some travelers are on business trips; others are on vacation. Yet, I can never tell the difference! Everyone is connected to a device instead of to the person right next to them. It is not healthy to take work on vacation. We need to give ourselves permission for downtime to rejuvenate. This means time not working *and* not thinking about work. Try to disconnect from email while you're on vacation; at least avoid mindless checking.

Finally, most everyone prepares with preemptive steps before leaving on vacation, such as enabling automatic email notifications and changing the answering machine message. But do you plan for re-entry? You want to avoid a crash landing! Don't be immediately stressed by returning to a full inbox on Monday morning. Block time on your calendar to catch up on emails and voicemail, even if that means working from home on your first day back.

I once had a boss who never returned from leave on a Monday. That was smart. Building in a transition period will allow you to regain a manageable work pace and workload so you don't feel overwhelmed. You'll avoid turbulence and have a smooth touchdown!

Mindfulness or Mindlessness?

Simply, mindfulness is the ability to focus. One must acquire the ability to appreciate what's going on in the present moment. If you think about it, there are three parts that we think about in our lives.

(Past) Rehashing: What we should have done, could have done, or would have done differently.

(Future) Rehearsing: What am I going to do tomorrow when I have that meeting?

(Present) Yet, the place where we have the most value and the most opportunity to transform our lives and our organizations is in the here and now. That's really all mindfulness teaches you to do: Be present and recognize the opportunities and challenges in the moment.

I want you to be in the moment and focus on what is real, here, and now. I want you to be listening to that patient's concerns. I want you to be in that meeting this afternoon and at the dinner table with your family tonight. I don't want you to be rehashing yesterday and worrying about tomorrow. After all, we have a finite amount of time. Make every day meaningful.

> *Yesterday is History.*
> *Tomorrow is a Mystery.*
> *Today is a Gift.*
> *That's why we call it The Present.*
>
> (Daft, 2016)

The Heart and Soul

Perhaps you've heard of the Big Rock Jar. Picture each day as a mason jar. People, tasks, and activities are the rocks that fill up the jar. We assign a large rock status to things with a higher priority. It's up to you to choose the largest, most important rocks and place them in the jar first. After the big rocks are in, then you can fill in the gaps with progressively smaller rocks and eventually with grains of sand.

However, if you put those less important things (the pebbles and sand) in your glass jar first, there won't be enough room for the big, important rocks. There's only so much room and everything will not fit.

Put aside solitary time for reflection and introspection to unearth what is inscribed on your big rocks. Do you have a close, warm emotional relationship? If you don't have someone special in your life, at least own a pet. (I could digress here, but pets seem to be able to give unconditional love, which is good for the heart and soul.)

What's in my mason jar? Paul, my soulmate and husband, close friends and family, pets, health, and well-being are a few of my biggest rocks. On the other hand, work is not a rock. Allow me to rephrase: Work is no longer a rock. It used to be a boulder. Now, it's more like a rubber ball. I can drop it, and it always bounces back!

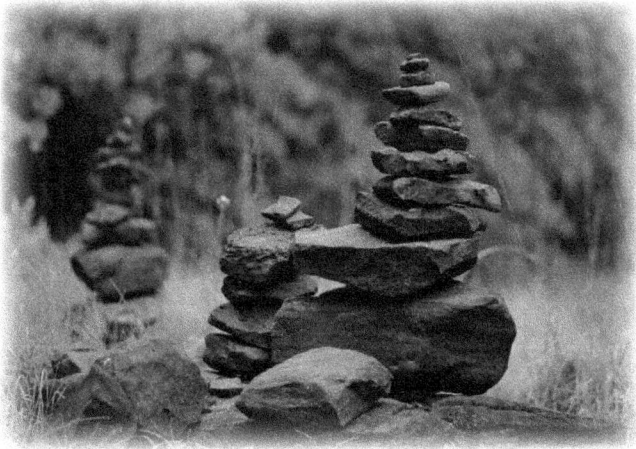

Caring for Others

Employee-centered organizations provide places of respite where workers can rest, relax, and reenergize by themselves or with colleagues. People perform their individual roles and collaborate better when they have opportunities to socialize and revitalize. Three suggestions on caring for others at work are provided below from simple to more complex.

Don't interrupt breaks unless it's absolutely necessary. Downtime is so important that you may be required by law to compensate employees for certain interruptions to their meal breaks. Meet with your director of human resources to discuss legal considerations related to meal breaks and compensation if you are unfamiliar with this topic.

A **Rescue Cart** for employees is similar to the concept of emergency crash carts used in hospitals to respond to code blue resuscitations. However, this unique cart is stocked with snacks, bottled water, books and magazines, personal care items, and other supplies to revive staff after stressful events. Provide stationery and pens for people to write notes of gratitude to fellow team members.

A cautionary note: the color of the cart should be distinct, such as purple, so it's not confused with emergency equipment.

People from several departments can share the cost and collaborate on supplies, design, and guidelines on use of the cart.

A **Quiet Room** is a restorative oasis to meet spiritual needs and provide relief from overstimulation. The area should be calming with neutral colors and soft lighting, uncluttered, close to a bathroom, and soundproof. Equip the space with a massage chair, water fountain, and selections of relaxing music and inspirational reading materials.

Healthy work environments promote positive patient outcomes. What can you do as a leader to promote rest and relaxation in the workplace? Ask employees for suggestions. My team recommended a pet therapy program. The implementation was labor and time intensive, but the therapeutic benefits for staff and patients alike far outweighed the effort. Moreover, it was a low-budget project since the therapy dog handlers volunteered their time.

Reflection

1. Use the rock image at the beginning of this section and write down a few of your biggest rocks.

2. List a minimum of five wellness and self-care activities. Include behaviors that help you to stay in good physical shape. Remember to also include activities in mental, emotional, and spiritual dimensions, particularly things that provide some sense of accomplishment. It may help to create categories based on time required or cost associated with each activity. In doing so, you may discover that you value relationships and time more than money and, similarly, experiences over possessions. You can earn more money, but you will never get more time. (Incidentally, "retail therapy" didn't even make my list, except to invest in good footwear.)

   1.
   2.
   3.
   4.
   5.

   Here are some suggestions from my list:

   Cutting down on stress by laughing. I enjoy watching a comedy or playing a funny game with friends.

   Going to a local center for performing arts on Sunday afternoons to watch my husband perform with the orchestra

   Watching hummingbirds and other wildlife

   Walking on a beach, or on a trail, especially with another person or a dog

   Gardening or engaging in creative hobbies

   Reading and writing

   Getting a pedicure or massage (without my mobile phone, of course)

   Wine (in moderation) and assorted hors d'oeuvres enjoyed by a warm firepit

   Short day trips, such as to the zoo or a museum

3. Keep the list handy in your locker or on a wall in your office as a reminder to care for yourself, too.

4. Next, choose at least one activity and make a goal to complete it within the next three days.

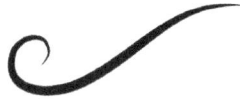

Domain Six: Lifelong Learning

Failure often lays the groundwork for success and it's only failure if we fail to get the learning.

Lifelong learning is the final domain in the model. Always strive to be learning something new. Do you remember the anticipation of graduation from your nursing program?

I once swore I'd never go back to school. Fortuitously, I later discovered that a college education is not the ceiling; it's only the floor.

We are at ground zero when we graduate and pass our boards. Initially, our focus is on developing competency—KSAs that give rise to behaviors needed for effective performance in our specialty. It's during this period that education becomes synergistic with work and experience. Combined, their effects are greater than individual parts. Concepts come together when learning is immediately applied on the job. We are now completing education and work with the same keystrokes and getting a double return on a single investment of time and energy. Knowledge builds much like compound interest.

The Journey

When we stop learning, the brain begins to atrophy and slowly dies. Likewise, when we stop developing, the same demise befalls our careers (Sandel, 2021).

A career-long learning continuum involves designing roadmaps (with technical, operational, and leadership content) that align with one's aspirations and goals for professional growth and development. It's no longer sufficient to be employable. You must also be marketable.

Foremost, avoid complacency. Always maintain an up-to-date resume so it's immediately accessible. Be diligent upfront in case a need or an opportunity unexpectedly arises. There may come a time when you must rescue yourself from unemployment during organizational downsizing and mergers.

Also, maintain a comprehensive curriculum vitae (CV) or portfolio. Just as artists have a portfolio of their works, you should create one of your leadership vision, attributes, and victories.

Indeed, there will be roadblocks and detours along the journey. Do your best to steer your career in the right direction and continually strive to bring value to your company. Look for skills needed to remain a beneficial contributor. With the advent of modern technologies, restrictions of contagious diseases, and other global concerns, education and healthcare are turning toward a new frontier. You cannot afford to remain status quo.

One can find himself obsolete in an organization due to rapid change. It's like being a deer in the headlights. You see a need to make a change; the danger is hurdling at you at sixty miles per hour, yet you are frozen in place. Some people lose their ability to respond to different ways of doing things. When this happens, they are plowed down. Maintain your ability to turn and pivot.

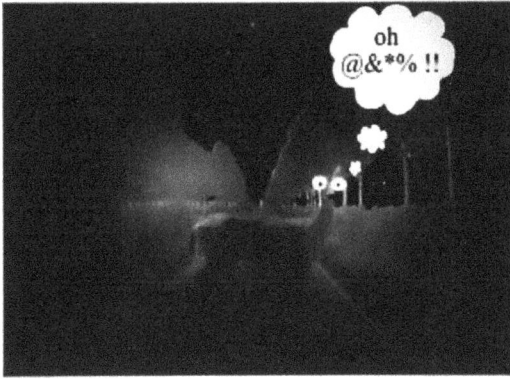

What happens if you accidentally swerve off course or run low on energy? Do you become lost, or do you refuel and get right back on track?

When we are weary, it's easy to lose motivation and our ability to focus on the road ahead. To stay driven and inspired, find something you love about your work and incorporate it into your schedule. Place it on your calendar as an appointment.

For example, I'm passionate about patient care and enjoy performing tasks, even if it's only starting intravenous lines. Find that one thing about nursing or your occupation that brings you happiness and make time to do it.

Other ways to recharge are by maintaining a spirit of inquiry, attending conferences, and participating in evidence-based, intellectual dialog like book clubs or blogs. You can begin today by starting ambitious yet achievable goals, such as continuing your education. Do you want to learn to play a musical instrument, begin a new hobby, or learn a foreign language? In the words of Spencer Coursen (2021), slow and up is always better than fast and down! You will discover that the more you focus on improving one area of your life, the more likely you are to enrich other areas of your life as well.

Naturally, bumps in the road and minor accidents are almost inevitable. Failure happens to everyone and is an opportunity to grow, learn, and improve. We can fail forward and learn from our mistakes.

It's often said that experience is the best teacher, and that might be true. However, it's not the best teacher if there is no learning; the outcome matters. After a significant success or failure, take time to reflect and learn what experience has to teach. Make critical self-reflection a new default.

Along the way, it's also essential to maintain some degree of technical and clinical proficiency. A nursing director once said it this way, "As your M for manager grows bigger and bigger, your S for skills shrinks smaller and smaller."

Our skills become rusty with a lack of practice. If I run into trouble when I'm trying to help at the bedside, I humbly request the nurses to "Please get your Ss over here stat!" (Ss meaning skills, of course!) Remember to maintain a record of your time spent in the clinical area.

Likewise, a practical suggestion is to maintain a daily productivity log to track all clinical and non-clinical activities. Tailor the document to your workflow, such as projects, meetings, and clinical hours. This is a tactical strategy in the event you ever need to justify your existence and show evidence of your worth. I've had bosses who required reporting to the extent that I needed to spend 20% of my time writing status reports. This micromanagement was counterproductive and a waste of time. Manage yourself and toot your own horn by delivering productivity reports without being asked.

Finally, the professional development of others is a personal passion for many leaders. The best supervisors focus on helping employees in their career development and progression. They work with their teams to develop action plans that focus on improving their employees' skills, abilities, and experiences. These leaders meet with direct reports frequently to discuss their growth and development. They have discussions about what is going well, what areas require improvement, and what support and resources are needed. The best supervisors are not selfish. They care about their people as much as they care about themselves.

Reflection

1. What is the one thing in nursing you are most passionate about? It doesn't need to be direct patient care. Your passion may be education or something entirely different that is also admirable and valued.

2. Is there anything you are mandating your team members to do that may be considered micromanagement or a waste of their time?

3. Develop a productivity log and time tracker to identify where you are spending your time.

4. Update your résumé and maintain a portfolio that includes certificates and continuing education credits.

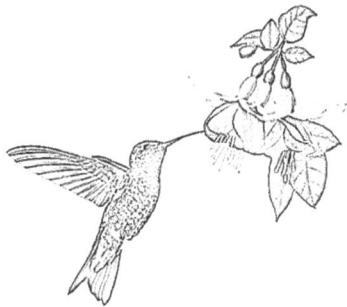

Chapter Three
What Gives Great Leaders Their Mojo?

As former First Lady Rosalyn Carter eloquently said, "A leader takes people where they want to go. A great leader takes people where they don't want to go but ought to be" (Goldin, 2018, para. 2).

How do we identify a genuine leader who knows when, where, and how to influence others? We certainly don't have to be appointed to a formal position of authority to lead. Personal power flows from individual knowledge, skills, competencies, and personality, not necessarily from the position held on an organizational chart.

There's not a comprehensive list of qualities all great leaders must possess. Everyone has shortcomings and blind spots. Most of us can identify distinct leadership qualities and behaviors, but without a doubt, that's the simple part.

The world is filled with self-professed leaders, people who spiel what they do not understand and endorse what they do not live. Understanding what to do is one thing. Doing the right thing can be quite another. Anyone who has ever tried to break a bad habit or lose weight can identify with this concept. The good news is that there are some leadership principles and practices that you can bank on along the way. All you need to do is mindfully act on them with positive intent.

In the following section, many components of the conceptual model, Domains of Success, are reiterated and linked with characteristics commonly associated with leaders. As you read, think of people whom you revere as leaders and identify as potential mentors. What makes them so inspirational? Make a note of the descriptors associated with leadership that resonate with you.

Putting It All Together: Leadership Characteristics

Morality: Most fundamentally, leaders cultivate integrity every day, and it's so pervasive that it becomes part of their DNA. Integrity is a steadfast adherence to a moral and ethical code. Unwavering moral commitment implies that we are consistent and act the same way in our personal lives as we do on the job. Behavior is not something you can compartmentalize into public or private life. Leaders cannot portray one face to a particular audience and a façade to a different one.

Further, never conduct an action that you wouldn't want broadcast in tomorrow's breaking headline news. We live in a hyperconnected world. Each action will have a consequence which may be positive or negative.

As in the words of Will Rogers, "Live so well that you wouldn't be ashamed to sell your parrot to the town gossip" (Handbook of Wisdom for Those in Transition, 2008, Quotation section, Will Rogers). Even a fleeting moment of indiscretion may place you in an unfavorable spotlight or surface instantaneously on social media. Everything is in a public arena for all to see and hear.

Moreover, whatever you put on the internet stays there forever. There is no such thing as "I deleted that." The costs of oversharing on social media can be very high. Our actions and interactions can either build or tarnish our reputation, impact future earning potential, and even influence opportunities for professional advancement. There's a consequence to every decision we make. Don't be scrutinized on the stand in the court of public opinion. The verdict may not be delivered in your favor.

We've seen myriad examples of people who have spent lifetimes building reputations and careers, and it only takes one scandal to lose everything. The higher we climb up the mountain, the more visible we become, and the peak is where lightning is more likely to strike! Integrity and honor cannot be like an alternating "off and on" current. They must be flowing like blood through your core at all times.

Similarly, people pay attention to everything a leader says and does. I didn't realize my staff even noticed (much less would remember) every word I uttered as a novice manager. It was not particularly constructive to think aloud and speak "off the cuff." Casual remarks twisted into the "gospel truth" and spread like a wildfire out of control. I'd spend the following days extinguishing the blazes.

A point worth remembering is that leaders are always on stage, so be a person worth watching and hearing. We are always representatives of our organization whether or not we are at the place of business, on a social media platform, or even on vacation.

What we don't do (our inactions) are just as important as our actions. Be a Superstar—not the subject of a breaking story on the six o'clock news or a "Firestarter" in your department. Consequences may be positive or negative, but every action has a corresponding ramification.

Just Behavior and Trustworthiness: Like honesty and integrity, other core values steadily guide a leader's decisions and behavior. Be fair-minded, equitable, honest, dependable, and always trustworthy. Trust doesn't come with a refill. Once it's gone, you probably won't get it back, and if you do, it will not be the same. Just like paper, once it's crumpled, it can never be perfect again.

Personality Traits: What about magnetism? Charismatic and motivational are terms frequently used to describe personalities of well-known leaders, but are these essential qualities? Similarly, is a leader's tempo always dynamic and energetic? The answer to both questions is that these attributes probably help but are not vital.

On the other hand, factors associated with emotional intelligence (EI) are necessary for effective leadership. According to psychologist and writer Daniel Goleman (2006), essential characteristics correlated with EI include self-awareness, empathy, and self-discipline. Goleman contends these factors can be cultivated and strengthened with immediate benefits to our relationships and work.

Visionary and Forward-Thinking Outlook: Leaders are visionary. Vision is an essential quality because it gives one direction and a picture of the desired future. Imagine someone giving you a 300-piece jigsaw puzzle with no instruction on what it's supposed to be. Could you put together the puzzle without the benefit of an image? Vision is very much like the illustration of the completed puzzle on the box.

People who operate without anything to guide them become frustrated, just as you would likely become in trying to piece a puzzle together blindly. A forward-thinking leader is innovative and capable of envisioning the future landscape and navigating the course to the desired future. Leadership involves shaping ideas and often changing how others think about what is desirable, possible, and even necessary.

Systems-Mentality Approach: Leaders operate from a systems' perspective and look beyond the functional areas for which they have direct accountability. The systems-approach is based on the premise that, in complex structures such as in healthcare, everything is interrelated and interdependent. Departments or subsystems cannot work solely in rigid, narrow-minded silos.

Individuals who operate from a systems-mentality also appreciate how their decisions and actions affect the entire workflow. Their goal is to optimize the performance of the organization or system as a whole. For instance, consider recruitment fairs and events where leaders rally to attract potential job candidates. A systems-thinker is not focused on recruiting talent exclusively for their unit of responsibility. Instead, the leader will refer qualified applicants to other areas in the organization if another department may be a better fit.

Agility in Chaos and Change: Today's leaders must also be agile and champion change. They must be transformational. Chaos and rapid reform are the new norms. What happens when the rug of normalcy is ripped out from underneath us? How do we react? Are we resilient and persevere? Or do we see unexpected situations, crises, and uncertainty as insurmountable problems?

For example, the Covid-19 crisis required adaptation to leading in a virtual environment. The walls of the old brick and mortar milieu came tumbling down. The pandemic has given rise to the prevalent use of telehealth due partly to federal waivers of Medicare rules authorizing eligible providers to use technology to deliver more services (Fauteux, 2021). Support personnel, such as information technology experts, are working remotely and cannot provide in-person assistance to frontline healthcare workers.

These challenging situations often present us with the best opportunity to learn who we are and who the people around us are. Undoubtedly, we will find shortcomings in ourselves and others, but we can strive to live up to the challenges. Leaders will emerge as innovators and proactive change agents, moving people in the right direction while getting them to do things differently.

Collaborative Qualities: Leaders realize they are a part of something bigger than themselves and are open to wisdom from wherever it may come, even unexpected places.

They understand no one is as intelligent as the collective whole. Diverse thought and different perspectives encourage creative solutions and lead to higher quality decisions, especially in dealing with complex problems. Matters of importance are viewed from as many angles as possible.

Team members can be corrupted by groupthink if we teach them to regard more highly those who think like them than those who think differently.

Leaders also know bringing out the best in others is how to find the best in ourselves and our teams. Just like in sports, if the quarterback focuses on making everyone else perform well, the team will be invincible. This means being more committed to the name on the front of the jersey than to the name on the back.

A leader is a supportive coach, placing others in positions to succeed while providing guidance and encouragement.

Decisiveness: Leaders can make hard decisions and often grapple with problems that don't have easy solutions. They don't rush to failure but, rather, confidently move toward excellence. In other words, leaders are reflective, not reactionary or reflexive (knee jerk). The analogy of a firefighter's job helps us understand the reactive approach toward work.

What do firefighters do? They sit in the fire station and wait for someone to phone in an alarm. They go to the location, put out the fire, then go back to the firehouse and wait for someone else to call in another alarm. This behavior is reactive, and it makes perfect sense in the context of the firefighting job, but it does not make sense in the case of leaders.

Think about reactive behaviors that leaders exhibit. When problems are presented at work, do you react to them only as they arise, or can you use them as opportunities to be proactive?

Teaching Talents: Great leaders are also great teachers but not necessarily in the traditional sense. They teach in diverse ways. One of the best methods to effectively develop others is by modeling behaviors. Great leaders are model organizational citizens and "walk the talk" by being engaged, enthusiastic, and positive.

Leaders also teach by knowledge-sharing, coaching, counseling, and one-on-one approaches with people they mentor. They do not squirrel away and hoard valuable information. We have a professional obligation to share our knowledge and work. Like a seasoned driving instructor, a leader functions as a guide without grabbing the wheel unless the situation is life-threatening.

Social Connectedness and Advocacy: Leaders cultivate robust personal and professional networks and healthy relationships. They do this not just within professional nursing organizations (although that's very important), but also in the business world and other entities such as government. Since the days of Florence Nightingale in the Crimean War, nurses have been the voice of advocacy for their patients. That's one thing that has not changed—nurses continue to positively influence healthcare politics and public safety on homeland and international fronts.

Expertise: Success as a leader is also linked to a wide bandwidth of knowledge and skills. Skills in receptive and expressive communication are critical. A respectable leader must also be intelligent, competent, and credible in an area of expertise. These qualities are needed to make sound judgments and decisions, as the story below illustrates.

As a new manager, I had a crash course in the cost of nonproductive time. I had recently taken over an emergency department struggling with productivity management. Charge nurses were not comfortable making staffing adjustments, such as flexing staff off early during low census periods.

One morning I walked in to find only a few patients, yet several registered nurses and technicians were sitting around the nurses' station. I asked for volunteers to clock out early. As luck would have it, an ambulance arrived with a critical patient shortly after we "right-sized." The staff could not obtain peripheral vascular access and needed extra hands. The charge nurse stormed into my office, brazenly poised with hands in the air, saying, "This is why we don't send people home early!"

I stood up from my desk, went to obtain supplies, and inserted an intraosseous (IO) needle on the first attempt. For those readers who are non-medical, IO access is the placement of a needle into the bone matrix and a very effective alternative to intravenous routes in emergencies.

The case was a pivotal moment in terms of gaining the respect of those present. Not only was I their leader, I was also a competent nurse who could be counted on. The team learned that I was willing and able to step outside of the management workspace and put boots on the ground.

Possessing a Business Acumen for Profit *and* Social Responsibility: Leaders must be organized with administrative talent, budgetary, and financial skills. Even non-profit organizations need a positive profit margin. After all, no margin, no mission! The organization must remain financially viable to meet its goals. Organizations face the reality of operating in a corporate context where there may or may not be shareholders, *but there will always be stakeholders.*

Leadership is a choice powered by a desire to make a positive difference, not only for today's stakeholders, but for future generations. Although business activity must focus on financial performance, it's not the only bottom line that must be considered. Organizational leaders must make a commitment to sustainability, which means to weave environmental and social efforts to preserve natural resources into all their decisions (Daft, 2016, p. 405). After all, there is no "*Plan*et" B.

No wonder leadership is scarce; it's so difficult! The challenge now is to transform our aspirations to be great leaders into reality. My friend Robyn once gave me a dish towel embroidered with pawprints and a motto. "Be the Person Your Dog Thinks You Are." That says it best.

Are you in it to win it? It's a lifelong journey. We never stop growing and learning. A good starting point for your journey is to create your own definition of a leader. I was inspired by Rosalyn Carter's perspective when I wrote what being a leader means to me. One may define a leader as a person of integrity who has the knowledge, skills, and ability to take people, not necessarily where they want to go, but rather to where they need to be in order to achieve the best possible outcomes even in the face of challenges. Now it's your turn!

Reflection

1. How do you describe a leader?

2. Who should be in your network?

3. Can you think of areas where stakeholder interests may conflict and you may find it difficult to concurrently satisfy demands of different groups?

4. Do you have a repertoire of knowledge, skills, and abilities necessary to lead in a variety of situations?

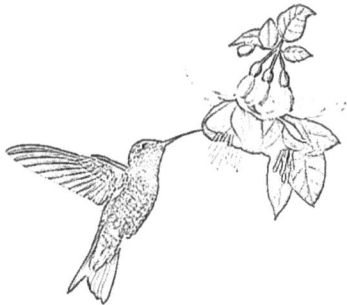

Chapter Four:
Management or Leadership? Be Ambidextrous!

Someone once said nursing leaders are not born—they are cornered!

In some cases, that may not be far from the truth. Several years ago, a chief nursing officer (CNO) Jeff rather abruptly requested that I step into an interim role as director of emergency services. He provided reassurance he would be with me every step of the way, and besides, the position was only for the short-term.

I knew from watching others that the higher we climb, the farther and harder we can also fall. After all, why was the former director's position suddenly available in the first place? I cautiously contemplated the proposal before responding with an affirmative answer. After several months of satisfactory performance in the temporary leadership role, I accepted a permanent title as the nurse manager—not director—in the same department.

I'm sharing this anecdote because, as a novice, I didn't understand there are demarcations between management and leadership. The terms are synonymous . . . or are they?

I was baffled when Jeff, stated, "You are functioning very well as a manager, however, not as a director."

He explained that management is a resource utilization skill and, as such, is fairly tactical. It entails control activities, planning, executing objectives, staffing and organizing, and performing other administrative tasks to maintain metrics within acceptable ranges.

An example of a control activity is evaluating the budget monthly and determining causes of any variances. Managers are in the best position to accurately determine the reason for a discrepancy. Monthly analysis can identify inefficiencies so remedial actions can be taken early if unfavorable variances are identified, such as in staffing. It is highly unlikely we will ever attain the exact expected volume, so we adjust staffing for our actual volume. However, by undertaking such timely reviews, we can better control results, so we come as near to the budget plan as possible.

As this example illustrates, the management role is essential for operations to run smoothly and efficiently, but it is not leadership. Transactional functions alone will not move an organization into the future. The organization will quickly become irrelevant if we only perform transactional tasks. The essence of authentic leadership is more ambiguous and transformational. It involves coping with change, extrapolating from the past, and creating a vision for the future because there is no steady state. You are either moving ahead or falling behind.

In his book, *The Power of Ted: The Empowerment Dynamic*, David Emerald (2016) describes the dynamic tension between management and leadership. It's true that management is focused on day-to-day operations whereas leadership is more closely associated being a person of influence, vision, purpose, and passion.

Yet in reality, we are pulled between these orientations every day. Management and leadership are different but complementary, and the roles often overlap. I unequivocally believe you can be a manager without being a leader, but you cannot be a leader without first being a good manager.

Consider someone who is trying to act as a leader but wants nothing to do with management. You may even know someone like this in your organization. I liken this to an adventurous eight-year-old who has located the keys to the family's SUV. He's overcome with a desire to drive to Disney World. Vision, a goal, a sense of purpose, and even passion are all present, but the ability to plan and execute is lacking.

I've worked with several individuals who wanted to lead but did not manage. They tried to explain themselves by saying they were visionaries and dealt best with the "big picture" things. I suppose they meant they came up with the ideas, but other people executed them.

These people may indeed have wonderful ideas, but without the ability to plan and oversee the necessary work, their ideas will never be realized—at least not by them. If their ideas are implemented, the work will be done by another leader who embraces the management function. Therefore, it seems rational to conclude that to be a great leader, one must be ambidextrous and function equally well in leadership and management roles. Do you concur?

Reflection

Fill in the chart with terms and short phrases under the most suitable heading as shown.

Leader	Manager
Innovate	Administer / Execute
Keep eyes on the horizon	Keep eyes on the bottom line

Focus on effectiveness vs. Focus on efficiency

Justify budgetary variances vs. Future resource allocation

Strategy vs. Tactics

Hands-on vs. Hands off

Softer skills vs. Processes and procedures

Hands on the wheel of the ship vs. Chart the course

Control systems and people vs. Inspires and leads

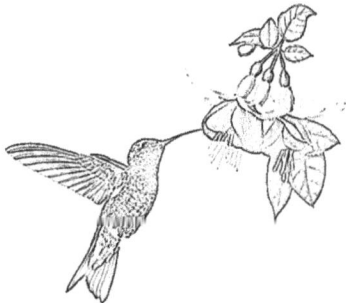

Part Two

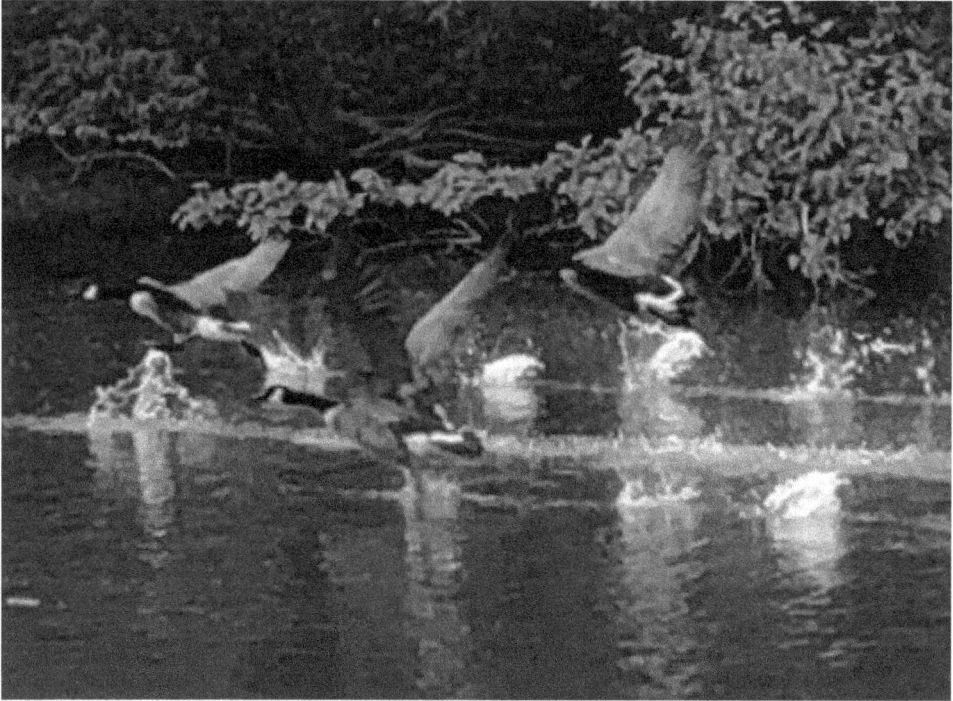

Chapter Five:
Day to Day Managerial Operations: The Nuts and Bolts with Tips and Tidbits

While we would all prefer to be in utopia—perhaps on a tropical Hawaiian island with our feet up and a fancy cocktail in our hands—the reality is most of us have to work. We spend a substantial portion of our lives on the job, so it's imperative we are happy with our work environment.

Yet, nurses are confronted with the daily reality of ever-changing corporate, operational, financial, and regulatory demands while in the relentless pursuit of excellent patient outcomes. Is it feasible, then, to create a legacy so one day you can look back and say, "I made a positive difference and truly experienced joy along the way?"

The answer is, indisputably, YES! Although you can't ride this ship alone, you can steer a course toward a better future, hold steady against the ocean's turbulent waves, and find happiness wherever you lay anchor. To begin, be open to wisdom and diverse ideas from wherever you find them. Don't be tugged down into the rip currents of mainstream thinking and indoctrination. Insights may very well come from unexpected sources.

Take geese, for example. I've discovered some of life's best lessons in nature, such as valuing the contributions of everyone.

Lessons from the Geese is a favorite and timeless parable used in many leadership programs, yet often without proper reference to its origin. Due to diligent research conducted by Sue Widemark, this composition is properly attributed to Dr. Robert McNeish. According to Widemark (2009), Dr. McNeish is a retired school administrator and a former biology teacher. He enjoyed birdwatching on Maryland's Eastern Shore and was intrigued by a brochure he picked up which gave many interesting facts about geese. He wrote the insightful metaphor on lessons from geese for a lay sermon he delivered in Northminster Presbyterian Church in Reisterstown, Maryland in 1972. The following excerpt is slightly modified from the original work with supplementary *postscripts*; however, the brilliant lessons are reverently credited to Dr. McNeish.

Lesson 1): Sharing a Common Goal: The reason geese fly in a classic V-formation is because the whole flock adds 71 % greater flying range than if each bird flew independently. As each goose flaps its wings, it creates an updraft for the birds that follow. The flock can reach their destination more efficiently by lessening wind resistance and conserving energy in this way.

People who share a common strategic vision of the desired future can reach their goals faster and easier because they are traveling on the thrust of one another.

Lesson 2): The Importance of Teamwork: When a goose falls out of formation, it suddenly feels the drag and resistance of flying solo. It quickly moves back into formation to take advantage of the lifting power of the birds in front.

If we have as much sense as geese, we will remain in line with those headed in the direction we want to go. We willingly accept assistance and offer our help to others.

Lesson 3) Shared Leadership and Empowering Others: Migrating geese share the leading position. When a goose inevitably tires of flying up front, it drops back into formation and another goose assumes the lead position. In essence, the lead goose becomes a follower.

Great leaders understand how and when to follow. They respect and support others' unique knowledge, skills, and abilities.

Lesson 4) The Importance of Empathy and Understanding: When a goose gets sick or injured, two geese drop out of formation and follow it down to the ground to help and protect it. They stay with it until it dies or is able to fly again. Then, they launch out with another formation or catch up with their flock.

If we have as much sense as geese, we will stand by each other in difficult times, as well as when we are strong. We will have empathy for one another.

Lesson 5) The Importance of Encouragement: Geese flying in formation honk to encourage those up front to keep up their speed.

We need to make sure our honking is encouraging and inspiring. Provide positive and constructive feedback, offer praise, and publicly reward good work. Productivity is greater and people are motivated in teams where there is encouragement.

Reflection

Before reading further, take a few moments to portray what utopia looks like to you. If that's difficult, then imagine a dystopia, and transform the description to an affirmative form, i.e., in dystopia, everyone works in silos, vs. in utopia, we have effective team dynamics.

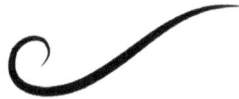

Empowerment and Delegation in Utopia

In utopia, there are ample opportunities for everyone's learning and development.

At one time I referred to human beings as "human resources." Heed a word of caution—people are not resources. They are our partners and colleagues. Empowerment is power sharing, as in the delegation of power or authority. Analogous to the geese, we should utilize others' capabilities, talents, and resources.

A well-known practice is to adopt a shared governance structure to engage organizational citizens in problem-solving and decision-making on issues that impact their profession and clinical outcomes. There are many reasons why participation in shared governance should be an expectation not an invitation. Foremost, frontline nurses know best how to make work processes safer, more efficient, quicker, more cost-effective with less waste, and of better quality. For example, as scientists were discovering ways to fight the Covid-19 virus, nurses were making innovations and thousands of adaptations every day on the frontlines of the pandemic (Dominis, 2021). Some nurses seized opportunities in telehealth. Others developed ideas to minimize the spread of infection, such as moving equipment toward the doorways of patient rooms. Nurses are finally getting the credit they deserved all along.

Moreover, empowered employees act more like owners than renters; they will do what is necessary and perform at their best to achieve excellent outcomes.

Delegation of power or authority is also a developmental tool, particularly when leaders invest time in training and coaching team members. Wise leaders understand that maximizing the potential of those who work for them is morale-boosting.

I'm forever grateful to my wonderful boss Linda who assigned projects that stretched my capabilities and comfort zone. Then, she always committed time and resources to remedy any knowledge deficits. She introduced me to the first version of Microsoft Excel® before it ever gained popularity. I've utilized and built upon this foundational computer skill throughout my career. It was interesting to learn the various software functions, and I advanced my abilities over time. Our work becomes more challenging and exciting when we practice new skills.

As it turned out, Linda was an enabler. The word *enabler* is not an insult in this context. A shared-governance organizational structure is where it's not only acceptable to be an enabler, it's desirable. As leaders, our job is to mentor and remove obstacles, then get out of the way and allow others to do their work. That was Linda's modus operandi. Yet, some people may avoid delegating because they feel it takes too much time, too much effort, or they don't know where to begin. Sometimes it seems easier to perform the task yourself and move on.

Nevertheless, in the end, delegation is a time-saving tool and will result in more freedom for leaders to work on higher-level initiatives.

Tips on the Art of Delegation

It's important to delegate purposefully and to follow a well-defined procedure just as you would when performing any skill. First and foremost, be aware of what you can and cannot delegate according to existing state laws, scope of practice, and organizational policy. Then, before you delegate, carefully determine the following:

- Who is going to do the task?
- Why is it appropriate for this person to do this particular task?
- Is the task associated with an area of interest or applicable to a scholastic project? (Delegation provides an excellent opportunity to help someone acquire skills on the job while earning academic credit.)
- Is the person competent to perform the task and has competency been validated, if necessary?
- What are the desired outcomes?
- What are your expectations?
- What do you want the person to learn from this developmental opportunity?
- What, if any, are the relevant constraints or barriers?
- How far can they go in moving ahead with the task?
- Is the task time-sensitive?
- Are there budgetary constraints?

- What are their boundaries of authority and responsibility?

Consider specific elements when creating an action plan. For example, an action plan for a committee appointment should comprise:

- Obtaining consent from committee members as outlined in bylaws prior to nominating an employee to represent your department.
- Adding the employee's name to group email distribution listings and meeting invitations, once the committee appointment is approved.
- Accompanying the employee to the initial meeting and delivering introductions.
- Scheduling the employee to work on the meeting days to avoid unnecessary travel to and from the workplace.
- Finally, dedicating time for the employee to attend the meetings, even if this requires that you place your boots on the ground to fill a clinical assignment for the duration of the meeting.

Meet with the employee to review the plan. As the leader, you remain responsible and accountable for actions or inactions of others in relation to delegation. Inadequate communication is the most common area for failure.

Don't get too mired in the details, but rather, emphasize the desired results.

Provide autonomy when possible. Instead of micromanaging, protect time for scheduled checkpoints and reporting. During these sessions, try to avoid the urge to immediately provide the solutions to an employee's problems; instead, use open-ended questions to analyze the best possible solutions. Naturally, it's easier to provide solutions, but instead, try to answer questions with questions to encourage critical thinking.

Finally, conduct a final review of the delegation. Provide feedback so learning can occur from the opportunity. This is a great occasion to have conversations with employees. This is also a great time to ask them for feedback on how YOU did a as a leader. Recognize the contributions of your direct reports and reward them for a job well done. As a bonus, delegated tasks may be linked to the annual performance review process with excerpts or short summaries from final meetings when projects are reviewed.

Reflection

1. List three tasks, projects, or meetings you can begin delegating.

    1)
    2)
    3)

2. Using the questions under **Tips on the Art of Delegation**, document the delegated task as an action plan. Consider creating a delegation log to track meetings and milestones for delegated tasks in a spreadsheet.

3. As a change agent, what additional recommendations would you propose on delegation?

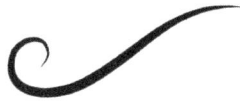

Change in Utopia

In utopia, there is an aura of stability even amidst constant change.
People drive change and embrace new technologies.

Leaders must be aware of how they react and respond to change. After all, change is ubiquitous in today's world of complexity and chaos, and the bulk of a leader's job is to facilitate the process.

As Charles Darwin reasoned, it's not the most fit of the species who survives, nor the most intelligent, but the ones most adept at handling change. Nevertheless, I believe the only people who *always* appreciate changes are babies in wet diapers! Most people prefer to maintain the status quo while hoping for continued success and an even brighter tomorrow.

Yet, hope is not a strategy. One cannot afford to stand by and allow a successful past to block the ability to foresee and anticipate the future. We have to keep pushing forward or we risk being left behind. As Holly Jackson (2020) asserted, we cannot become comfortable and ride on past achievements! Fortunately, there are many techniques and approaches to dealing with change.

Most current research builds upon classical work conducted by a German-American psychologist Kurt Lewin in the mid-1900s. Lewin developed a widely accepted archetype of change theory: unfreezing, movement, and refreezing or "cementing" the change in place (Marquis & Carol Jorgensen Huston, 2000). Although there are numerous strategies and theories for leading change, there are also many common denominators. The purpose of this section is to review several general concepts related to successfully leading change initiatives.

Having a high-quality idea is never enough. These two critical first steps to leading change go hand in hand: 1) creating a sense of urgency and 2) helping others understand a change is required. Urgency is a vital first step to help employees move from feeling content with the status quo to seeing the importance of changing sooner rather than later. Yet, be aware that creating an aura of urgency is not the same as inducing stress and anxiety. People affected by the change need a clear and compelling reason to move out of their comfort zones, and as a leader, you need their acceptance for it to be successful. Paint a realistic picture of the reason for the change. For example, don't protect employees from troubling data or dangers lurking behind the decision for a change. To borrow a term from Lewin, a leader must unfreeze the current state so employees are motivated to invest the resources required to adopt new techniques, processes, or procedures. The need for change must outweigh the resistance to it, and it must resonate with all. A leader must share a clear vision of a desirable future and reassurance that the organization is on the right path at the right time.

Good leaders also communicate the vision early with those most involved and affected by the change. Never let your employees find out about a change from outside sources! Communicate often and in a variety of ways; employ all available channels of communication. Break announcements down into small, manageable parts while keeping key individuals informed on the reasoning, facts, and direction of changes. Halt the rumor mill by encouraging team members to ask clarifying questions rather than conjuring up specious conclusions.

Similarly, it's crucial to acknowledge emotional concerns throughout the course of change. When people ask questions, be respectful and don't assume they are being resistant to change. I was sometimes negatively labeled as resistant when I was simply trying to learn a little more in order to become comfortable with what I was being asked to do.

Training may be required to help people understand and cope with their roles in the change. Employees should thoroughly understand the change and its influence on them. Excellent leaders encourage participation which will foster acceptance.

Establishing a coalition to guide the change and including a variety of people are keys to success. Involve people who will be impacted by the change as well as those with enough power and influence to drive the change process. Utilizing volunteer change champions who are deeply committed to the change will foster results. Value and tap into the diversity within your organization for different perspectives and plurality of ideas.

Create small successes and leverage wins along the way by placing focus on some easily attainable goals. Celebrating wins will reward the people involved while building momentum. Like the geese, maintain the thrust and honk to offer praise and reward good work.

Don't stop the change movement before it is hardwired and sustained. Establish benchmarks, then monitor compliance to assure metrics are moving in the desired direction.

Update all relevant systems, policies, and processes to support the change.

Later, don't sit idly by waiting for the next change. I promise: another change is lurking just over the horizon. Be a trailblazer. By taking hold of the reins and pursuing change, you will create an opportunity for yourself and your team. And please, don't be a sieve who blocks ideas from brewing and coming to fruition. Many creative ideas are filtered by middle managers and never percolate up to the C-suite for due consideration. Strive to develop a workplace where innovation, new ideas, new ways of thinking, and new working methods are ingrained in the culture. Keep riding the horse in the direction it is going or get out of the saddle.

Reflection

Think of a situation at work or in your personal life that involved significant change. I recall events, such as the conversion from paper to electronic documentation and major organizational restructuring in the forms of downsizing and mergers.

1. What emotions did the major change induce?

2. What techniques were used to make the change possible?

3. As a change agent, what additional recommendations would you propose?

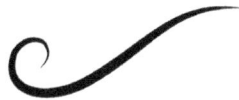

Management and Organization

In utopia, operational and administrative processes are highly efficient. Even email is manageable!

How often do you carry unfinished work home because there are not enough hours in the frenzied workday? Even worse, have you ever taken a sick day only for the opportunity to work in solitude without disruptions? As a manager, the only time I didn't haul work home was after a grueling twelve- or fourteen-hour day. Every Sunday night, I would boot up the laptop and work on payroll to meet the Monday morning deadline. Work bled over into my family and social life. My computer and briefcase were constant companions, even escorts who chaperoned every vacation.

Fortunately, life experiences are better now as I continue to exercise my attention-management muscle. Note I did not use the phrase *time management*. Attention management is the practice of controlling distractions, being fully present, finding flow, and maximizing focus (Thomas, 2018).

Time management is nothing more than a myth. There are only twenty-four hours in a day. No more, no less. All we can manage is ourselves and what we do with the gift of time we're given. Rather than being derailed by distractions, we decide where to direct our attention based on priorities. In other words, we should be intentional instead of reactive.

The following strategies may be helpful if, like me, you sometimes struggle with finding enough time in your day.

Take back control of your time and priorities. Print your calendar at the start of each workday or try visual management with a dry-erase board. YOU choose where to direct your attention.

Remember to delegate. Tap into underutilized talents.

Place a clock on your desktop or wear a device so you can easily track time.

Keep a notepad and pencil handy to jot down notes.

Control your environment. Set boundaries with others. Schedule and post office hours to decrease interruptions or even go to another part of the building such as a library when you need uninterrupted time for a project. When interrupted, we don't go immediately back to our peak performance level. It takes a while to work back to optimal functioning. Employees are typically willing to wait, and you will avoid disruptions if you have dedicated time for drop-ins. Team up with your colleagues to designate a no-distraction or quiet hour for focused work on priority projects or quiet solitude for incubation of ideas.

Use single-tasking. Give your undivided attention to a single task. If you think of something else that requires attention, jot it down on your notepad and come back to it later. A helpful technique is to focus on your task for twenty-five minutes, then take a five-minute break. Repeat this cycle four times, twenty-five minutes of work and five minutes off. Then, take a twenty-minute mental break to stretch, hydrate, or take a short walk.

Bundle tasks and limit motion. For example, if you work in a large building, get organized and manage as many tasks as possible in a single trip to avoid walking back and forth between your office and other departments. Not only can this incessant trudging be physically taxing, but it's also wasteful. When you print a daily calendar and task list, you can spot ways to bundle activities and make time-saving changes to your schedule.

Keep your workspace organized and uncluttered. Handle paper only once. Try the WAD approach to paper: WAD it up (wastebasket, action, delegate) or file it.

Make the most of wait times. Carry a notebook and paper, book, or other reading materials in your briefcase for productive activities during delays.

Control your technology. It is there to serve you, not vice versa. Distraction is always just a thumb-swipe away. If you spend much time watching television or surfing the web, then a valuable hack is to minimize idle distractions. Email, discussed next, is another area where you may uncover more time-saving opportunities.

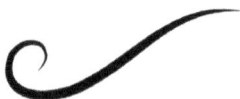

Netiquette and Email 101

We live in an age of digital deluge, constantly inundated with a flood of incoming text messages and emails. These interruptions can easily veer us off course, or even worse, we can become overwhelmed and drown in information. Have you ever checked text messages in face-to-face meetings (although it is impolite) or attempted to multi-task by perusing emails while talking on the phone? If so, then try closing the floodgates by implementing the following key strategies.

Create boundaries. Schedule specific times for checking email, only two or three times a day. Know your high energy periods and own that time for projects and work that requires creativity, like writing. I own the morning. Don't waste the most productive part of your day sorting and deleting emails.

Reduce interruptions. Turn off the notification feature for when an email comes across. If not, each prompt will be a trigger and tempt you to glance at the message. You can quickly take the bait, become hooked, and get reeled in.

Use tools to help manage and organize mail. These tools include flags and folders. Flag an email message to remind yourself to follow up at a later time. Use folders to make it easier to find messages. Many programs have a method for differentiating emails received from individuals you identify as very important people.

Limit information that you do not need to receive and limit the messages you send. Try alternatives to traditional email responses, such as creating a poll and using voting buttons. Be considerate of others' time and avoid the dreaded reply to all. Use the unsubscribe feature for junk mail. An email should not be the default form of communication. For every email you send, you are likely to get two or three back. A former boss and highly regarded vice president of operations once told me he limits emails to three in any given chain. After that, he shows up at your door or picks up the phone.

Proper grammar and netiquette are also essential considerations. Email is a form of social interaction. It's a reflection of who you are and how competent you are. Be polite. Don't use email for therapy; it's not a forum to vent. Never send a message when you are angry or continue a dispute via email. Simply, don't start an email war! Sensitive issues are better handled face-to-face.

Similarly, be careful not to misinterpret the written word. We may not read an email or text message correctly and that can guide a set of inappropriate actions that can have a domino effect. Email is missing so many signals and lacks instant feedback such as facial expressions, eye contact, body language, and voice tone. Words are all we receive in written messages and sometimes people misinterpret intent. Give correspondence from others the benefit of the doubt and request a face-to-face encounter. The same VP of operations also taught me, "When in doubt, assume good intentions." You might say, "I interpreted your email this way . . ." It may simply be the person who sent the email is not aware of how the message is received, and you've misinterpreted the message because of the writer's style.

Explain the nature of your message in the subject line.

Express your intentions clearly and concisely.

Do not rely solely on computer spell check. Someone once submitted a job application and noted "Candy Stripper" as relevant volunteer work experience in a hospital. (No, I will not disclose the facility's name where she performed these services.)

Never use all capitals because it may be interpreted as shouting and rude.

Avoid using red and red underlines (reserve this for editing).

Avoid emoticons in business communications. You may do this with friends, but this is not professional in business communications. Likewise, limit the use of humor because it can come across in an unintended manner, even cynical. Also avoid inappropriate acronyms like OMG and inappropriate greetings like *hey*.

Imagine what your email would look like projected on a courtroom wall. Remember writing is permanent. Think and pause before you post. It may be helpful to read the email out loud to hear what it sounds like before you hit the send key and the message is in the cloud forever.

Reflection

1. List three strategies you can implement to better control your time at work.

2. Activate two computer functions to make email more effective and powerful. Ask members of your IT department for their expertise and suggestions.

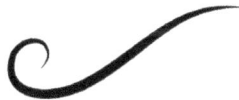

Meetings

In utopia, we have fewer meetings because we are so darn good at them!

Did you list fewer meetings as a strategy to control your time at work? There were days so consumed with meetings that I didn't get back to my office until five in the afternoon. I squandered away many hours in unproductive sessions. On some days, I sat in my soft leather chair with high earning executives around the table and pondered, "How much money and how many resources are we collectively wasting just by virtue of being assembled in this room?"

Over the years, I've learned tactics that give rise to constructive meetings that people look forward to attending. The relative success depends on what occurs at three distinct junctures: what happens before, during, and after a meeting.

Before the Meeting

Communicate the primary purpose in advance of all meetings. Always try to let people know why they have been called to a meeting to eliminate speculation and avert fear of the unknown. It's troublesome to get an early morning call from administration requesting your presence in the CEO's office later in the afternoon.

Worse still, imagine being telephoned by a receptionist regarding a mystery appointment with the director of human resources. It's even more nerve-racking when the meeting is scheduled on a Friday just before the close of business and you are denied an explanation.

What do you think was on my mind the rest of the workday when this happened to me? I was unable to focus on anything else. Later, at the end of a seemingly endless day, the mystery was solved. When I met with the director of human resources, she apologetically informed me the payroll department uncovered an error during an audit. I was entitled to back pay with interest as compensation and received an unexpected check on the spot. Get the point? The anxiety was rational and normal, but was it necessary? As an executive leader, would you handle this situation differently?

Provide agendas in advance of meetings with a clearly stated purpose and desired outcome(s). Here's an example.

Purpose (The Why): Fulfill a mission opportunity to bring better health to the underserved by reaching beyond the boundaries of our brick-and-mortar building in the provision of healthcare resources to the broader community.

Desired Outcome: Increase access to primary and preventative medical care for uninsured adults and children by providing mobile health services in the community by the end of this fiscal year.

Additionally, when sending agendas, direct participants to prepare in advance of the meeting, such as to read policies that will require their approval. It's unsettling to ask for a motion to accept a policy followed by a period of uncomfortable silence and the realization that no one has bothered to read the document beforehand. It's disrespectful and a waste of everyone's time. Voting on a document you neglected to review is a form of social loathing and displays a dangerous lack of individual accountability. Vital details can fall through the cracks. You may be the only expert at the table with a piece of critical knowledge related to a policy or procedure.

For instance, clinical nurses are likely to be more knowledgeable than the chief nursing officer (or anyone else in the room) on the numerous intricacies involved in the process of safe drug administration, such as the use of dispensing systems, scanning techniques, and the operation of various equipment like pumps. The people who do the work are best equipped to recognize and solve the problems. Don't be the missing link that results in a deadly, yet preventable error.

Remember to notify individuals with pre-assigned roles, such as the timekeeper and recorder. Most people dread the responsibility of recording minutes, so assign this task on a rotating schedule. As a planner, you have the unique ability to make it easier for the recorder. Before the meeting, use the agenda as a blueprint for recording the minutes. Utilize headings for each topic on the agenda, then insert key, pre-determined discussion points to decrease the amount of notetaking required in real time.

Finally, it's always a good idea to have a little book or collection of reflections close at hand during all gatherings. I've been in many assemblies where the leader asked for a volunteer to offer a devotion. Be the person who is ready to offer a meaningful reflection.

Here's a favorite from my collection that is especially pertinent during the present-day Covid crisis.

A Reflection on A.S.A.P.

Ever wonder about the abbreviation A.S.A.P.? In our line of work, we think of it in terms of even more urgency and stress. As Soon As Possible. Perhaps, if we think of this acronym in a different manner, we will find an uplifting way to deal with these challenging days.

There's work to do, [many demands] to meet,
[more and more patients to see and treat.]
But as you hurry and scurry,
A.S.A.P. - ALWAYS SAY A PRAYER.

In the midst of [crises and] chaos,
"Quality time" is rare.
[Just] do your best; let God do the rest:
A.S.A.P. - ALWAYS SAY A PRAYER.

It may seem like your [cares and] worries
are more than you can bear.
[Pause and take a deep breath, and]
A.S.A.P. - ALWAYS SAY A PRAYER.

God knows how stressful life can be;
He wants to ease your cares,
And He'll respond to all your needs
A.S.A.P.- ALWAYS SAY A PRAYER.

An adapted version (Reflections in the WORD, 2010).

Just before the meeting, arrive with enough time to ensure the room is properly set up. I've walked into meeting rooms and found chairs strewn about, leftover food, dirty dishes, and empty coffee carafes. You may need time to tidy up. Complete an audiovisual equipment check and adjust lighting. Be prepared to greet participants as they enter.

During the Meeting

Begin the meeting by establishing ground rules. For recurring meetings, print the ground rules on every agenda for review at the beginning of each session. These are the participants' rules, not yours. Offer one or two examples to get started, then hand the floor over to the attendees.

Examples of Proposed Ground Rules:
    Begin and end on time.
    Seek common ground and understanding.
    Stay on topic.
    One person speaks at a time, and everyone has a chance to
        talk.
    Be present.
    Avoid back-channel discussions during meetings; instead,
        bring relevant or value-added information to the
        surface for all to hear.
    Respect the view of others.
    Check understanding by asking questions.
    Listen to understand, not to contradict.
    Constructive, honest debate is desirable.
    Attack problems not people.
    Silence implies agreement.

Some meetings are an opportunity for recognition, such as to present service awards or express appreciation.

Throughout the meeting, acknowledge employees who contribute by asking clarifying questions or offering good advice.

Great leaders also make it the norm to talk about elephants in the room. Is there support for participants to speak the unspeakable within your organization? Are you aware of issues that need to be addressed but nobody is ready or willing to discuss? As a leader, take time and make it safe to talk about those hard things everybody is thinking, but no one is saying.

Next comes an even more difficult component. Offer everyone a platform to share opinions. It's an excellent strategy to withhold your point of view until other team members have had a chance to first express their point of view. I acknowledge that asking for other perspectives can be difficult. Sometimes, you just don't want to hear pushback, especially on a personally developed idea or plan. Yet, the stakes are not in your favor if people are not willing to give you honest feedback.

Be prepared to be challenged and make changes. Surround yourself with people who exercise independent judgment, who are willing to say something different from their leader's perspective and test assumptions. Don't let notions of hierarchy get in the way.

Don't interrupt but do paraphrase during pauses to let participants know they are being heard and to clarify key ideas. Paraphrasing also provides an opportunity to ascertain if you correctly interpreted what was said. After soliciting feedback, the next step is to acknowledge and act on recommendations.

Everyone wants meetings to end on time, especially right before lunch or at the close of a business day! There are a few proven techniques to keep meetings on track.

Negative polling is a time-saving tool that can be utilized during the closing part of a discussion to determine if the group is ready to confirm a decision and move on to the next topic. It is sometimes easier to reveal disagreement within a group than to confirm agreement. When using this tool, the leader can simply ask if there is anyone in the group who cannot agree with what has been suggested or put forth by participants. If no one speaks up, it is generally acceptable to move on.

When a discussion gets off track and participants are talking about issues that are not on the agenda, ask everyone to pause and reconsider the meeting purpose or desired objectives. As chairperson you may say, "I sense this issue is important to many of you but is not the purpose of our meeting today, so may we table this discussion until a later time?"

Utilize a flip chart page or ask the recorder to keep a sheet labeled "Parking Lot." Sidetrack items are placed in the parking lot and reviewed later to determine if any should be included in a future agenda. The leader will need to follow-up on all questions and issues recorded in the parking lot.

A final concern is how to manage disruptive behaviors. Ignoring disruptive behavior will adversely affect members of the group and their perception of your leadership. Have you ever been in a meeting where people were silently imploring the leader to contend with a disruptive person? You might say, "Let's see if we can address your concerns as we move forward. If we can't, then let's discuss it during our next break."

Another common technique is the Situation-Behavior-Impact (SBI) Technique.

> Step 1: Describe the situation and behavior. For example, "Paul and JoAnne, you have left and returned two times since the meeting started."

> Step 2: Make an impact statement to explain how their actions are affecting the leader, the process, and other attendees. For example, "We had to stop our discussion and start over twice because of this."

> Step 3: Redirect the person's behavior. This can be done by asking for suggestions about what to do. For example, "What needs to happen to ensure this does not happen again?" Or you may ask, "Would the group like a short break so that when we return everyone will be able to fully participate?" This sounds like parenting, but then leadership is sometimes like parenting.

After the Meeting

Following these guidelines should deter meetings after the meetings. I'm referring to the water fountain griping, grumbling, and complaining that sometimes occur in clusters outside a meeting room. Unfortunately, these gatherings can be more impactful than the meeting itself.

The hallway is not the place where people should vent their opinions and shape decisions. Unfortunately, if the guidelines we discussed are not adhered to, then the hallway may be perceived as safer than the boardroom.

Finally, promptly follow through on any action items to which you commit. Allot time to review and distribute minutes (ASAP). It's best to complete record keeping immediately following the meeting for easier and more accurate recollections.

Virtual Meetings

Like it or not, most everyone is forced to experience virtual meetings as a participant, a leader, or both. In my experience, virtual meetings can be very dry, and often there is minimal downtime for social interaction to talk about things unrelated to work. Gone are the days of bumping into a colleague in the break room or going for a brisk team walk around the building. What can be done on the virtual front to boost morale and build team cohesiveness during this time of social distancing?

The internet has myriad cyber games and activities from ice breakers to fitness sessions. My favorite is a Bring Your Pet to Work Day. Another suggestion is to invite an employee's grandmother to join a video call and share insights from what her world was like several decades ago. As a child, I learned some very valuable lessons while sitting at the feet of my elders. The older I get, the smarter my grandparents become. You can even arrange to have batches of homemade cookies delivered to homes or offices for everyone to enjoy during the call.

As a final note, mute phones during conference calls. Background noise is annoying to co-workers and infringes on your privacy. Careless comments are uncomfortable for the group and may be embarrassing or even fast-track your career in a direction you don't want it to go. The reflection exercises that follow are designed to help you prepare for your next successful meeting.

Reflection

1. In the role of a participant, suggest a minimum of three ground rules for a meeting.

2. Locate a resource for daily reflections such as a John Maxwell book, or begin to create your own collection.

3. Search the internet for virtual games and ice breakers, and try one during your next cyber meeting.

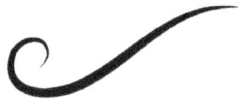

Tools and Equipment

In utopia, we have all of the tools, supplies, and equipment required to perform our jobs.

The Gallup organization is infamous for its World Poll, but did you know the company is also in the business of research and corporate consulting services, including an acclaimed employee engagement survey known as Q12?

As the title implies, the survey consists of twelve workplace items or questions that offer an empirical link to performance outcomes. The focus of this discussion is the second survey question (Q2): "Do you have the materials and equipment to do your work correctly?"

Question two is highlighted because our team didn't fare well on this item for two consecutive years, and I learned a valuable lesson worth sharing. Discouragingly, the mean score failed to improve from one year to the next despite all my best efforts.

On the subsequent survey, people reported they *still* didn't have the tools and equipment needed to perform their jobs adequately. Somewhere I had made an oversight. On the upside, I recognized that the key to dealing effectively with a blunder is to embrace it, learn from it, and then share lessons learned to build competence throughout the organization. So, I began by conducting a post-mortem to solve the mystery. I was amazed by what I learned.

Anatomy of the Q2 Error

I discovered the genesis of the debacle began with a faulty assumption, "The manager knows best." (To my credit, I grew up watching *Father Knows Best*, a classic television program that is telling of my age.)

So, I attempted to fix the problem single-handedly. First, I met with the director of finance, and we earmarked sizable capital expenditures for state-of-the-art equipment, stretchers, and monitors. It

106

sounds like a boss's dream come true, right? It was like Christmas every day of that year! But, instead of boughs of holly, I decked the halls and rooms with high ticket items like cutting-edge gadgets, more bells and whistles, and new tools.

Then, we repeated the survey the following year. I eagerly anticipated the Q2 results and envisioned a world class percentile ranking. Yet, my prediction was flawed and wide off the mark. The Gallup Q2 was one of the lowest scoring items in the report. By the way, this is a day that I received a call to meet with our chief nursing officer in administration to discuss the survey results. I didn't have answers (at least not yet), but I did shoulder all the responsibility for the results.

In despair and frustration, I scheduled a staff meeting to review the survey results. Each employee received a copy of the report. I professed that I didn't understand the crux of the nursing issues related to tools and equipment. After all, we were one of the few departments privileged to receive capital funding from a limited pool of resources. We should be appreciative, correct? Weren't we blessed with more than our fair slice of the pie? So, what went wrong?

I was flabbergasted by the simplicity of the answer. Nurses told me they needed a coat rack at triage so people wouldn't place their coats and handbags on the pediatric scales. They wanted more bedpans and urinals. A late-shift weekend technician shared the desire to have the same access to supplies (catheters, fluids, and tubing) as the day shift people after the storeroom is restocked on a Monday morning.

The nurses and technicians expounded on their frustrations, such as reaching for a patient care item at the point of care and discovering an empty bin. Then, walking down the hall to the supply closet and finding no one has replenished the par level.

Nightshift workers have only three options when supplies are depleted: improvise, call and wait on the nursing supervisor to obtain the required items, or leave the department (and patients) to meet security personnel at the storeroom to locate supplies in a hunt and find fashion. The result is inefficient resource utilization, extended patient visits, and low staff morale. It's also a safety concern when staff members leave their patient assignment to track down equipment in other departments.

Whether it's positive or negative, feedback is always a gift and critical to a leader's success. Based on comments from staff members, I graciously asked for volunteers to develop an action plan. A clinical care leader, the director of material management, storeroom personnel, nurses, and other staff members formed a committee to optimize supply levels. The committee recommended an inventory management method using barcode technology. The team also determined the minimum amount of stock to always have on hand so that an automated message is electronically transmitted to the storeroom when stock numbers drop below the par level. Additionally, storeroom personnel were scheduled to evaluate inventory on Friday afternoons.

For my part, I began to listen and implemented a stoplight method to help manage equipment requests. The tool is a living document composed of five columns with a key to provide meaning of each color.

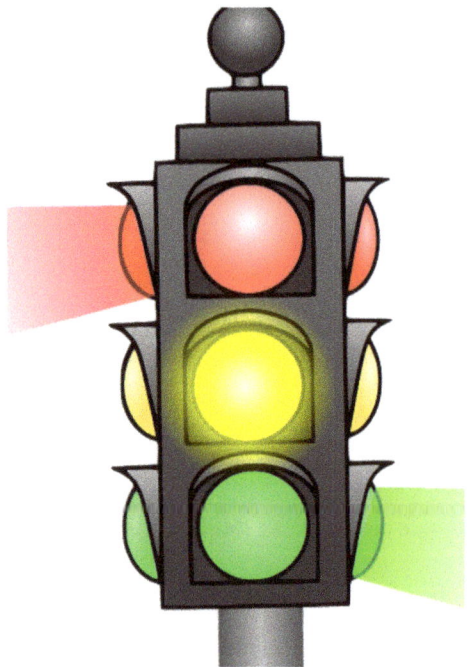

Columns
1) Tools and Equipment (items requested)
2) Source of Request (for follow-up and recognition)
3) Stoplight Color (red, yellow, or green)
4) Notes/Updates
5) Cost

Key

Green: complete, equipment purchased and requisite installation and training complete

Yellow: a work in progress with status notes, such as on back order or budgeted

Red: not able to grant request but with explanatory notes to provide rationale for denial

I used the stoplight method to provide updates on requests during daily rounding, via emails, and in the weekly newsletter with recognition to everyone making suggestions.

Remember to give feedback to people who took time out of their day to communicate a need. Let them know, "Got it, thank you! I will come back and ask you questions as needed." Along the way, inform them about progress made on the recommendation. Think about it; if you needed a new piece of equipment and shared your idea, but then you heard nothing about it, and you talked to your colleagues, who said, "Oh yeah, I gave an idea, too, and I haven't heard anything," eventually, the spigots are going to be turned off. It's not even going to come through as a trickle. If people don't think their ideas are valued, then they are going to stop giving suggestions.

The following year we were world class! I was invited to the company's convention to share the *team's* success story in a presentation to hundreds of leaders. In leadership, when everything goes right, you give away all the credit to the team, and when everything goes wrong, you take all the responsibility.

Reflection

1. Create your own stoplight form and try this method over several months.

2. Utilize the tool during rounding and share the living document with your team as it is edited and updated.

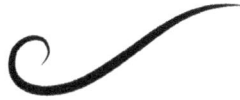

Tips on Presentations

In utopia, public speaking is rewarding and energizing, especially when it's about your team's success!

Glossophobia is a riveting term for fear of public speaking. A large proportion of the populace share this affliction. Leaders are not immune. Most everyone has suffered anxiety, dread, and apprehension at one time or another when taking center stage to speak before a crowd of onlookers. Some even shy away and avoid speaking engagements altogether.

Yet, the floodgates of opportunity open for those few who put forth the extra effort required to become outstanding presenters. Advantages include increasing your earning potential, more effective personal and professional networking, catapulting employment opportunities, broadening recognition, and many more. So, don't gloss over your potential. The journey to becoming an extraordinary presenter can begin here and now.

A starting point is with the book *The Exceptional Presenter* by Timothy J. Koegel, a well-thumbed reference in my library and a highly recommended resource. This quick and easy read provides tips to improve your presentation style, most notably using the acronym OPEN UP.

But, before reading further, take a moment to write the names of two admirable orators, such as a politician, preacher, professor, or perhaps an acquaintance in your organization. Then, list four attributes that describe each of their presentation styles.

Name:	Name:
1.	1.
2.	2.
3.	3.
4.	4.

The Meaning of OPEN UP—Much More Than Letters

Through years of inquiry and research, Koegel developed a winning formula that transforms mediocre presenters into exceptional presenters. He discovered the secret is to OPEN UP with this key:

"O" is for Organized: Exceptional presenters are organized with a well-designed and clear message. Begin with the end in mind. What is your purpose? To inspire action, to teach something, or perhaps to change perceptions?

Utilize a prep form as a blueprint to arrange your presentation and include notes, such as audiovisual needs.

The format is very important. Koegel reminds us of a timeless structure:

1) tell them what you're going to tell them (the opening frame)

2) tell them (the body which is structured with an outline, and

3) tell them what you just told them (the closing)

"P" is for Passionate: Exceptional presenters exude feelings of passion for their topic. If the presenter is not excited about the subject, why should anyone else be? As the adage goes, "People don't care how much you know, until they know how much you care" (Koegel, 2007, p.96).

The audience will undoubtedly sense if you lack genuine enthusiasm because passion cannot be contrived. You can scream, jump up and down, and all around the stage. That's just too much expresso. So, if you're not passionate about the topic, then the first task is to find some emotional association to what you are presenting so your passion naturally gleams through.

"E" is for Engaging: Exceptional presenters are engaging and easily bond with the audience. Practice telling a story in the opening. I strive for edutainment (education + entertainment) to maintain attention and engagement when the presentation aims to teach a concept. You may even consider instilling humor with relevant video clips to help convey key ideas; however, don't rely too heavily on technology. Props, such as flip charts and markers, can be strategically placed around the room to encourage audience participation in meetings. Sometimes small tokens and rewards, such as a meal or lottery ticket, can engage the audience and encourage responses during events.

"N" is for Natural: Koegel ascribed the final letter in OPEN to remind us to have a natural, relaxed presentation style. We've all experienced those exceptional presenters who appear comfortable, eloquently speaking in conversational tones with a captivating voice and enchanting eye contact. In essence, they own the room, making it appear that giving a presentation is easy to do, enjoyable, rewarding, and energizing!

If OPEN is an acronym for being organized, passionate, engaging, and natural, then what's UP? According to Koegel, exceptional presenters must also "understand the audience" and "practice."

"U" is for Understanding the Audience: Put effort into preparing to speak to issues and concerns that are meaningful to your audience. Doing homework beforehand will pay big dividends.

It may be as easy as picking up the phone and calling to inquire about significant points of interest. It has also served me well to mingle with participants just before giving a presentation. Making personal connections puts me at ease. Valuable morsels of information gleaned from informal chats, such as recent impactful or celebratory events, can be woven into the presentation.

"P" is for Practice: Naturally, presentations must be rehearsed. Practice, practice, practice! It takes dedicated time and repetition to master new skills, but the return on investment can be significant. If you don't practice, you will not improve your ability to deliver effective presentations. Leaders are always in the spotlight and center stage, so there are plenty of opportunities to polish presentation skills.

Reflection

1. How did the characteristics you listed at the beginning of this section compare with attributes in the reading on OPEN UP?

2. Find an opportunity to present a topic of interest and ask trusted colleagues for objective appraisals. Provide worksheets for their assessments and include basic categories, such as:

   Was the presentation organized?
   Did I come across as passionate and engaging?
   How was my posture? Voice? Eye contact? Facial expressions?
   Did I eliminate verbal graffiti? (Um, you know, I kinda guess
       what I really mean to ask is if I sounded good, okay?)
   Was the delivery natural and conversational?
   Request the appraisers to rate the presentation on a scale
       from 1-10.

3. Review the critiques and keep practicing! You will not always be perfect. Blunders will happen, so it's best to practice daily instead of waiting until the stakes are high. As Abigail Van Buren is credited with saying, "If you want a place in the sun, you have to put up with a few blisters."

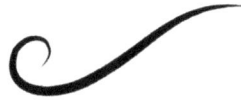

Performance Improvement

In utopia, we are never satisfied with the status quo.
While others are resting, we are striving for continuous improvement.
We spare no effort when it comes to being world class because we care.

Is there anyone or anything at work you find particularly annoying? I am easily frustrated by information sieves in any form—humans included. Allow me to explain.

Sometimes innovative ideas for improvement are already within an organization amongst employees who are closest to the customers. Frontline workers often know better than anyone else how to get their jobs done, and make processes more efficient, safer, faster, and cheaper, and deliver a higher quality product. Yet, 51% of employees surveyed by a Harris poll reported that managers often make poor decisions because employee knowledge is not utilized (Daft, 2016). I don't want employees leaving their brains behind in the locker room when they come to work. Do you?

So, why is it that middle managers underutilize this readily accessible, free resource and block creative thoughts from percolating to the top echelons inside their organizations? Two reasons come to mind.

First, it's common knowledge that many people, some managers included, don't like change. The second reason is frontline managers

114

may feel so overwhelmed with the daily grind that they don't allocate time for improvements and innovation. Does this ring true?

On the other hand, the best leaders seek to make a difference by searching for improvement opportunities, taking action, and persevering until they bring about meaningful and sustainable change. Moreover, these leaders don't operate in a vacuum. Instead, they leverage experiences of older workers and fresh perspectives of new hires alike. These trailblazing leaders teach us to embrace diversity and be mindful that everyone comes to our team with different but valuable insights. Moreover, they drive momentum and know it's necessary to take reasonable risks.

Things won't always go smoothly but the best leaders are tenacious. It's not, "If at first you don't succeed, try harder." Instead, it's, "If at first you don't succeed, try something different."

In simple terms, unhook and try a different approach. Remember, in the end, what you want to look at is not only what you changed, but the difference it made—the outcomes. Strive to develop a workplace where innovation and new ways of working are a part of the culture.

Performance Improvement Strategies

You don't need to become a performance improvement (PI) specialist to be a great leader. Still, I recommend that leaders at all levels become familiar with various PI methodologies, such as Six Sigma or PDSA (Plan, Do, Study, and Act) and participate in group projects, such as Kaizen events designed to improve processes. You can even practice performance improvement strategies like PDSA or 5 S: Sort, Set, Shine, Standardize, and Sustain at home. The experimentation can be fun. You may even save money!

To illustrate a simple Do-It-Yourself (DIY) application of the PDSA problem-solving method, we will examine a problem most everyone has experienced. Assume you want to decrease your monthly electric bill. First, quantify the amount of expected decrease in energy consumption with a range of variability and develop a plan. What types of changes can you and your family implement to minimize the utilization of energy? Think of a few ideas to pilot on a small scale that suit your unique situation. Keep it simple.

For example, if you have children (or a spouse) who will not turn off lights, then you may decide to invest in motion sensors or timers that turn lights on and off automatically. Perhaps you thought about changing old bulbs for the newer, more energy-efficient ones. Maybe you decide to tweak the thermostat and lock it in the new setting. The important thing is to develop a good *Plan* and define the length of time you will work the project in the *Do* phase. When you review the results, determine if the decrease is what you expected, or do you need to alter your plan and go through another cycle of improvement?

In this example, you will want to monitor the electric bill every month, collect, and then analyze data over time. This is the *Study* phase. Keep notes. A single checkpoint in time, such as one billing cycle, will not provide sufficient data to inform your decisions. Make comparisons to prior bills in the same time period and consider variables such as unseasonal fluctuations in temperatures, such as record highs and lows.

In the *Act* phase, determine what you learned and identify necessary modifications. You may decide to adopt the changes because you are getting results that meet your expectations. If the performance results are not what you expected, then what else can you do? You can adapt or modify the changes that were made and then rerun the plan, do, study, act cycle again. Or should you abandon the changes? Perhaps you actually need to replace your windows and augment insulation or invest in solar panels.

Lean is another PI approach for optimizing workflow. The desired outcome of any Lean project is to deliver value to the customer by efficiently producing quality end-products that are precisely what they need, when they need it, and in the quantity required using minimum resources (i.e., materials, equipment, space, and time). The focus of this brief introduction is limited to the identification and elimination of waste. Further study of Lean methods and principles is highly recommended.

Waste Not, Want Not

Any form of waste is problematic because it does nothing more than impede flow and degrade value. From the consumer's view, waste adds zero value. The acronym DOWNTIME is a helpful tool for recalling tips and tidbits for easy recall of wastes. Grant yourself permission to take some "downtime" to identify examples of waste while you become acquainted with the eight common categories presented below.

D for Defects or Do-over is the rework needed to be done in a process not done correctly the first time. Errors also fall within this category, as when nurses inadvertently provide discharge instructions and even prescriptions to the wrong patients. In addition to obvious safety concerns, giving information intended for someone else has other significant consequences.

For example, we know the Health Insurance Portability and Accountability Act of 1996, commonly referred to as HIPAA, sets standards for privacy of protected health information (PHI). The accidental disclosure of an individual's PHI is a serious and potentially litigious matter. An organization can incur damaging publicity and financial penalties for breaches. A tremendous amount of time and resources are used in mitigating the effects of a single breach. I've even traveled for hours to retrieve PHI from private residences!

As a manager, I was frustrated and in dire need of an error-proofing solution. I turned to the "KISS' EM" approach: "Keep It Safe, Simple, Effective, and Manageable" for a fail-safe way to eliminate the defect. We tweaked the discharge process by highlighting patient identifiers, such as name and date of birth, on all discharge forms together with the patient or responsible party for confirmation. My director, Amy, recommended a catchy phrase, so we termed the new process "Highlight to Get it Right!" The slogan was easy to recall and even appealing. If properly followed, this procedure makes it nearly impossible to disclose the wrong patient's information. The bulk purchase of 64 highlighters was less than $25.00. On the other hand, the monetary penalty for HIPAA non-compliance can be as high as $50,000 per occurrence (HIPAA Journal, 2021). You choose.

O for Overproduction is where an organization produces more than what is necessary, and it's one of the worst offenders because it leads to deficiencies in all the other categories.

As another example, consider an antiquated practice of routinely drawing a rainbow of labs (collecting extra blood tubes of every possible color) just in case the vials are needed for add-on laboratory studies at a later time. The rationale is it expedites additional lab work (add-ons) and prevents subsequent venipunctures.

This practice is wasteful, and the actual benefits are low (Snozek et al., 2019). Besides, medical practitioners abandoned the practice of bloodletting in the early nineteenth century, and only the leeches complained.

W for Waiting is where either a person, an operator, or a machine is waiting because there is a delay in the process. No one pays to wait. All veteran emergency nurses know that nothing good ever happens in the waiting room!

N for Non-utilized talent is any time we have human capacity or creativity not being used. Tap into the talents of individuals within your organization. Also, cross-train people to help each other perform a variety of functions rather than having people trained to perform only one particular task. This helps to balance the workload and allows for flexibility.

T for Transportation is where there is a lot of unnecessary movement. Why transport a patient to the main treatment area when they can be seen and treated closer to triage?

I for Inventory can be raw material, finished goods, or money held in reserve that doesn't need to be held in reserve. There are many, many forms of inventory, and all of them are pretty much wasteful.

M or Motion is when there is excessive motion of the operator or the machine. This example involves physical motion of people. I worked in a department where we had to walk to another section of the building to take documents off a central printer. The purpose of a shared printer was to save money. The concept appeared logical and efficient at first glance, but the bean counters failed to factor in the manpower time, interruptions, energy, and frustration involved in leaving the office (maybe locking the door) and traveling to the remote printer. Habitually there would be an issue with the printer requiring multiple trips between the office computer and printing machine. The end users were not consulted on the change to a centralized printer, so this serves as another example of why it is important to seek input from the people who do the work.

E for Extra Processing might be in the form of extra sign-offs on contracts or other superfluous steps. One example is the arduous process of policy approval where it can take months as documents slowly progress through committees, oftentimes with setbacks in the form of revisions. Many organizations hurt themselves with slow decision making. The Lean method can be utilized to streamline the policy approval process and eliminate analysis paralysis in decision making. After all, a well analyzed problem does not solve the problem.

Don't Be Data Rich and Information Poor

No discussion on performance improvement is complete without reference to data. Even though we live in an age of data deluge, metrics alone do not drive our behavior nor stimulate action. Therefore, it's essential to tell the whole story when reporting numbers. Simply reporting figures to your staff will not get you the results you want.

For example, blood culture contamination rates can be reported month after month, but the percentages are meaningless unless phlebotomists understand the value (the *why*) for decreasing contamination rates. Always begin with the *why* and then describe the *how* and *what* parts of the work.

Likewise, when you are asked for data (and this will be very often), it's helpful to ask how the data will be used. If the information will be used to solve a problem, then you may be able to help create a solution rather than just regurgitating data. It costs money and time to collect and report data. Don't perform non-value-added activities that impede efficiency, such as unnecessary reporting. Measure what you value and explain the why.

Reflection

1. Here's one way you may be able to spot opportunities for improvement. Lay down on a stretcher, close the curtain or crack the door, and use your senses to see, feel, and listen. Look at the ceiling. Are you comfortable? What conversations can you hear? Ask at least two staff members to do the same and compare results. After doing this activity, a staff member recommended we install fluorescent light covers with peaceful scenes designed to reduce anxiety or provide distraction.

2. Visit your organization's Performance Improvement Specialist(s). Does your leadership team apply a particular methodology for performance improvement, or are various strategies employed depending on the project size, complexity, and type? Do you have an ambitious team member interested in performance improvement projects and serving on a PI Committee?

3. Name three examples of waste in your department.

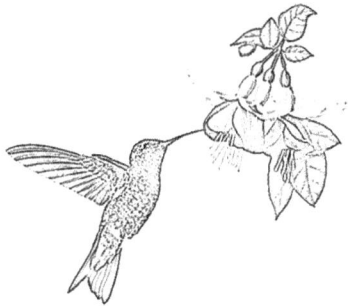

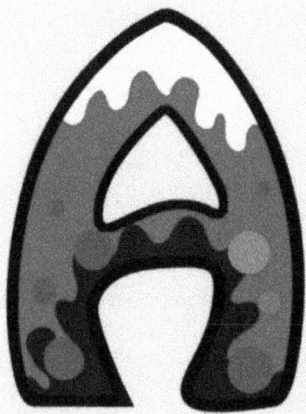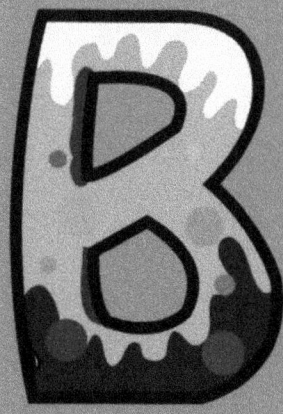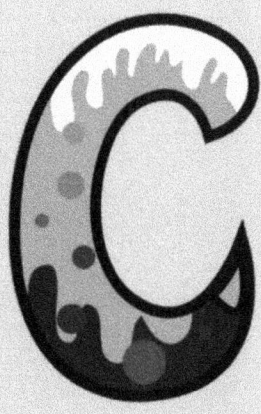

Chapter Six:
Human Resource Operations

Train employees well enough so they can leave; treat them well enough so they don't want to.

To be an effective leader, one must be aware of Human Resource (HR) principles, including all relevant policies and procedures. Otherwise, you'll likely make promises you can't keep or deal with situations inappropriately only because you don't understand the correct approach. It would be best to have a great HR mentor or partner—someone who can straightforwardly tell you what you can and cannot do and whether you're doing the right thing. It's wise to always follow basic HR rules.

In this section, an introductory review of selected HR principles prefaces attention to three specific managerial functions: hiring, performance appraisals, and crucial conversations. Information within this work is not intended to constitute legal advice. The guidelines and other subject matter are intended for informational purposes only.

Basic HR Guidelines

Whether you're an experienced leader or a novice, a good rule of thumb is to work closely with HR to ensure compliance with U.S.

employment laws and regulations, such as those set forth by the Occupational Safety and Health Administration (OSHA) and U.S. Equal Employment Opportunity Commission (EEOC). You don't need a law degree to be a great leader, but you do need sufficient knowledge to steer clear of potential litigious pitfalls and protect against employment lawsuits. Also, be aware state laws on discrimination may be more stringent than federal laws, so always seek expertise.

Likely you are already familiar with some mandates such as Equal Opportunity requiring employment decisions to be job and business-related and not based on race, ethnicity, gender, age, pregnancy, religion, military/veteran status, and other factors.

However, employment law is complex, and the language is as mixed-up as a hearty pot of alphabet soup. Here's a spoonful to sample: FMLA: Family Medical Leave Act; BFOQ: Bona fide occupational qualification; ADEA: Age Discrimination in Employment Act; ADA: Americans with Disabilities Act of 1990 and ADAAA: ADA Amendments Act of 2008; FLSA: Fair Labor Standards Act; and PDA: Pregnancy Discrimination Act. The pot seems bottomless. The point here is not to frighten anyone, but to stress the importance of the first two HR guidelines:

1) When in doubt, always seek expert advice BEFORE acting.

2) Keep abreast of changes and complete annual education on the subject of HR issues. There are several additional guidelines leaders can follow to guard against legal predicaments.

Discipline can be used as an example. Employees will notice if a manager is not performing appropriate disciplinary actions. Infractions, such as tardiness and absenteeism or disrespectful behavior to superiors and coworkers, damage the work environment, harm the employer brand, and decrease workplace productivity. A lack of discipline can be an irritant to high performers.

Regardless of your personal feelings toward an employee, your behavior must be fair and consistent. Any deviations will quickly become apparent and undermine the perceptions of the leader's objectivity and employees' trust. In the extreme, failure to apply rules consistently to all employees may even be grounds for a legal finding of unjust action and trigger financial penalties. Hence, the next guideline.

3) Incorporate HR review of all grievous corrective actions to ensure discipline is consistent with similar historical cases and does not violate union contracts, employment, or other laws, organizational policy, or cultural norms. For example, if someone has to be fired, then you want HR to say, "Yes. Everything is in order to proceed."

We want the termination process to be humane and effective. Correspondingly, it's also critical to understand and respect employees' rights. Do not retaliate or in any way interfere with an employee exercising rights and privileges, such as in making appeals, contacting HR, or engaging in any other legally protected activity, such as calling an employee hotline.

Before moving on to the fourth guideline, consider a rhetorical question. Have you noticed some people are engaged and with you from the start, some sit on the fence, and still others will never be with you - no matter what you do? Don't waste much time on this last group. As a novice manager, I wasted a great deal of time on the latter disgruntled group without any return on the investment. Frankly, there was collateral damage when good employees separated. If only I had followed guideline number four.

4) Direct attention to the engaged and committed employees. Employee behaviors directly influence individual and business performance. A shift in focus to engaged employees will result in better retention and customer focus, fewer mistakes, and increased productivity and efficiency.

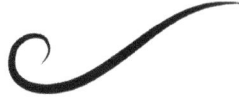

Additional HR Guidelines

5) Read your Code of Conduct handbook. If you don't own a copy, obtain one today. Also, maintain documentation that all employees received, read, and understand the Code of Conduct and have access to a current employee handbook.

6) Utilize the Employee Assistance Program (EAP). You are not qualified or capable of solving your employees' personal problems.

7) Assure all references are up-to-date and all forms are current.

8) Process employee actions, such as terminations, promptly.

9) Maintain thorough documentation. For example, track dates in real-time as leave is taken utilizing FMLA.

10) Off-boarding separated staff members is as important as onboarding new hires. Be attentive to timely completion of administrative tasks, obtaining ID badges, and notifying departments to delete access to computer systems and drug dispensing machines. A checklist is a useful tool to create for this purpose.

11) Remember to contact your risk manager or attorney to obtain counsel for any legal questions, concerns, or issues.

12) Treat employees as people who have feelings and reasons for doing what they do. Get to know your employees and understand their reasoning. You might learn something new.

Reflection

1. Who are your resources (names and titles) for consultation on difficult employee issues?

2. Review your organizational code of conduct. Assure all employees have access to the employee handbook and code of conduct.

3. Create an off-boarding checklist. Include sections for the name of your department, supervisor's contact information, employee name, ID number, termination date, and a checklist of essential tasks and notifications. Confer with HR as you build the tool and share the form with other leaders.

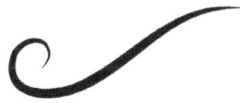

Avoiding Self-Inflicted Injury from Employee Turnover: A Prophylactic Approach

Hiring new employees is a significant investment in terms of time, resources, and money. A conservative estimate of the cost associated with replacing a separated employee ranges from one-half to two times the individual's annual salary.

Costs per hire comprise advertising expenses, referral incentives, screening costs (such as background checks), recruiter salaries, miscellaneous fees, such as for testing and post-hire orientation. Other costs don't register in black and white on a productivity report. For example, turnover can negatively impact team morale and burden other employees with an increased workload. A continuous stream of new hires through an organization results in employees continually climbing the learning curve rather than performing to their full potential. Then, when employees finally begin to function at an optimal level, they may be recruited by a competitor. Some people haven't learned the grass may look greener on the other side, but it still must be mowed!

Give some forethought to the necessity of requesting new positions and consider if you can reorganize or improve processes in ways other than hiring. Also, don't overlook the advantages of recruiting internally. Positive aspects of promoting from within the organization include historical company knowledge, organizational understanding, recognition for achievement, successful succession planning, and boosting employee morale while inspiring others.

Yet still the question remains, how can we stop the bleeding and stabilize the workforce? To do nothing to control the hemorrhage out the backside will eventually result in organizational demise because, as nurses know, all bleeding eventually stops. However, you will need more than a Band-Aid approach.

A favorite maxim is to Hire Hard and Manage Easy. The importance of hiring cannot be overstated. Don't just employ warm bodies; having a pulse is not enough of a qualification.

A philosophical issue to consider is whether to hire for competency or to hire for organizational cultural fit. When a company employs for organizational cultural fit, they consider individuals whose attitudes and values match theirs. When hiring for competency, they focus on an individual's skills, competencies, and experience.

It's important to consider both and maintain a balance. Even the brightest people may not fit in with the enterprise. You don't want to fall into the trap of hiring for competence only to later have to fire because the person does not conform well with the organizational culture. Employees who assimilate into an organization's culture tend to be more engaged, motivated, and collaborative. The likelihood they will remain productive, long-term employees increases, which adds value for all stakeholders. Remember, you can fix lack of skill but not lack of will.

We can provide training on new technology, processes, and procedures, but motivation and attitude are much harder to teach. To this end, I recommend two categories of interview questions. The first focuses on relevant knowledge, skills, and abilities; the second concentrates purely on cultural fit with questions aligned with organizational core values. Remember, the person you hire today is someone you may have to live with for years to come. However be prepared—this may mean rejecting applicants with the requisite technical skills.

For this reason, assuring a cultural fit should not end with the interview. Assist new employees in forming a connection with your organization's mission and purpose. It's not enough to hand them a booklet or project a slide with the company's mission and vision statements.

Often a flood of new information and materials are presented in a short time during organizational orientation. You need to help the new hires connect the dots, digest, and internalize what is most important. For example, if community-centered care is part of the mission, then schedule a time during orientation for the employees to see this in action. They need immersive experiences to live the values, not to simply rattle them off by rote memory. In the following section, a personal anecdote is shared to convey the power of a good cultural fit.

I recently had an eye-opening experience from the perspective of a daughter while visiting my mother Doris in a Florida hospital. While beautiful murals adorning every hallway, a classical pianist in the lobby, and fine furnishings made the visit more pleasant, any healthcare system can decorate a lobby. The decor is not what was important.

The people working in the hospital were the reason the experience was extraordinary. When a worker said hello to a guest in passing, you got the impression they *really* wanted to say hello, not that it was a mandate. Some organizations enforce the ten-foot rule, which requires employees to engage customers within ten feet. That was not the case here.

There is a coffee stand in the lobby of the hospital with 24-hour-a-day service. One early morning, I went to purchase a cup of java (actually, a venti, one-half 1%, the other half non-fat, extra hot, split quad shots with two shots of decaf and two shots regular brew, no foam latte, with whip, two packets of granular sugar, one sugar in the raw, just a touch of sugar-free vanilla syrup, and two sprinkles of cinnamon please). The complexity of my order could have tried the patience of Job, but I was served by a very kind and patient barista named Alix. When I asked Alix if he liked his job, he replied, "I love my job!"

He described how supervisors came by throughout the night shift to ask how he was doing and if there was anything he needed to do his job better. And not just his supervisor dropped by—even the nursing supervisor!

Next, Alix revealed a secret. He was also employed in a competitor's hospital on the other side of town for his day job. In this different position, supervisors tried to make sure employees did everything right and catch them doing something wrong. Alix said when he worked at this other job, he kept his head low and wanted only to get through the day to get a paycheck.

Quite to the contrary, when working nightshift at this hospital, he could be himself and found joy in working. This was the same person, but he engaged with his customers in two completely different ways.

Then why is it we, in leadership, are always saying how we need to get the right people on the bus? The reality is it isn't the people; it's the leadership. A leader's role is not being in charge. Instead, it's taking care of those in our charge. If leaders create the right environment, a utopia, we will get people like Alix at this hospital. If we create the wrong environment, a dystopia, we will get people like Alix at the other hospital. Which Alix do you want to work for you?

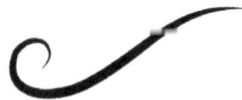

The Art of Interviewing and Hiring

My best recommendation on interviewing and hiring is simple: invest time in training yourself and your team of interviewers. Don't fall victim to dangerous legal pitfalls, like being accused of trying to ascertain ethnic background, country of origin, religion, gender, marital status, age, sexual orientation, or other prohibited information in an interview.

I observed unfortunate consequences when an inexperienced manager innocuously asked a male job applicant why he chose a nursing career. Frontline managers and team members who perform peer interviews must be acquainted with laws pertinent to the interview process.

Another suggestion is to partner with the talent consultant assigned to your area. After all, you share similar goals related to personnel. Talent consultants are held accountable for vacancy rates and first-year turnover. Recruiters work off generic job descriptions; they aren't mind readers. As leaders, we must communicate what we want and need in a candidate. Attend job fairs and other functions, such as visiting local universities to broaden your pool of suitable candidates.

Although not directly related to interviewing, be aware recruiters make an offer for a position before informing other viable applicants they were not selected. Your preferred candidate may not be willing to accept the job offer, so you need to keep others in the pipeline.

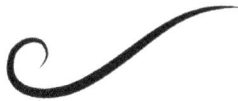

Interviewing Do's and Don'ts

Do maintain the dignity of the candidate.

Do be consistent and treat all candidates in the same manner.

Don't rely on first impressions. You've likely heard the simple premise to trust first impressions and gut feelings. I can't entirely agree because both positive and negative first impression errors occur, such as when a candidate is late for an interview. We must go beyond first impressions.

Do realistic job previews so candidates know what it's like to work in your department and what challenges they will face. Failure to be factual can be costly in terms of early resignation or termination. Be specific when possible.

- The job requires you to report to duty at 0645 and sometimes work late. Are you able to do that?
- This job requires working every other Sunday. Are you willing and able to do that?

Do consider shadowing and observation experiences as part of the interview process.

Don't stereotype! These are some common biases and stereotyping:

- Halo Effect occurs where one strong attribute overshadows all others.
- Horn Effect happens when one judges a candidate negatively based on one bad trait.
- Similar-to-me bias, such as "Oh, I went there, too!"
- Nonverbal biases, such as the pen clicker or another annoying interview behavior due to nervousness

Do allow silence, if necessary.

Do talk with people and get input from others who were not a part of the formal interview process. How did the interviewee interact with people they didn't believe would provide information, such as maintenance workers, environmental service personnel, registration clerks, or others?

Don't mislead applicants by using phrases such as great job! Instead, say something like, "Thank you. It sounds like the situation worked out well for you."

Don't make an assumption, such as someone with several children will miss time from work. They may truly have excellent time management skills. And what about an applicant with no children? The childless applicant may not disclose how he cares for his elderly parent who happens to live a hundred miles away.

Do collaborate with a mentor to develop questions in advance of interviews. Don't try to wing it! Relate questions to the job and job requirements.

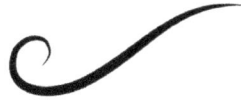

Behavior Predicts Behavior

As you develop interview questions, a simple premise to keep in mind is past behavior is the best predictor of future behavior, so ask behavioral questions. Obviously, the past is not an absolute predictor of the future, but it's a better indicator than intuition. One simple technique is known as STAR.

S - Situation
T - Task
A - Action
R - Results

The candidate describes a situation or task from his past, actions related to the event, and the results. Listen for what the applicant did. Use questions like these:

1) Describe a time when your team or organization was undergoing some change. How did the change impact you, how did you adapt, and was the change successful?

2) Give an example of a time you faced a conflict while working on a team. How did you handle the disagreements?

These questions focus on specific behaviors and skills necessary to be successful in a particular role.

Lastly, there are many reasons to invite staff to perform peer interviews, such as improved retention, buy-in, leadership development, and employee engagement. Invest in training staff members on the legal aspects of interviewing. Carefully select who will participate in peer interviews and include someone from the shift and in the same role the candidate has applied for, such as a unit secretary on the night shift.

Reflection

Using the STAR technique, write a minimum of two behavioral questions to use during your next interview.

1.

2.

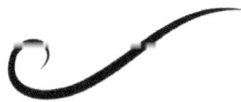

Post Hire

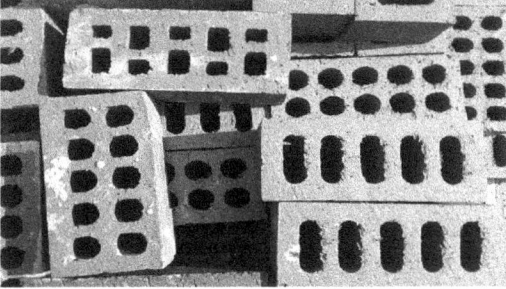

You've done all the hard work of screening, interviewing, and hiring, and finally, your new employee comes in excited and engaged. Yet, this will all come tumbling down like poorly laid bricks in a wall if you don't construct and sustain a solid foundation.

You can have excellent talent attraction techniques and still blunder as employees enter the door. Treat your new staff members like customers. Meet with them at the beginning and the end of their first day on the job. Take them to lunch. Partner with the professional development coordinator/specialist or educator, and the HR representative in planning orientation.

It's disconcerting how many organizations fail to deliver the essential resources and amenities on day one, such as a clean office or cubicle and equipment needed to do the job. Be attentive to the small stuff like a fresh coat of paint, email access, voicemail, ID badges, lockers, and business cards. There are stories of people who have had to function for days, weeks, and sometimes months before they had all the essentials.

A new boss once presented me with keys to an office littered with grimy file cabinets overflowing with a predecessor's sensitive files and personal items. I spent my first day cleaning and purging file cabinets. On the bright side, it didn't feel like a day at the dealership buying a new car and filling out form after form.

To prepare for employees, customize an onboarding checklist with elements essential for a stellar new hire experience. It's not a solo activity; partner with other areas of your organization to create a broad range of onboarding experiences, formal socialization, and networking. Something you can quickly implement is a NEWS Program or New Employee Social Hour. The NEWS Hour is an informal one-hour session for new hires to meet and share thoughts on what is going well, what could be better, and make meaningful social connections. It also provides an opportunity to attain an early resolution of concerns and to address questions:

How do I . . .?
Where do I find . . .?
Who do I call about . . .?
What is the policy on . . .?

The NEWS Hour is also a golden opportunity for positive molding and enculturation. Participants should include an HR representative, manager or director from any department, and professional development coordinator or educator. Additionally, executive leadership support is vital for a successful program.

For one NEWS Hour program, I paid out-of-pocket for refreshments because the chief nursing officer wouldn't approve a stipend for coffee and refreshments! I suppose she favored the high-ticket expenses of turnover more than the cost of a dozen donuts.

For new leaders, schedule a meet-and-greet social hour with members of the leadership team. Provide all new employees with learning opportunities to understand how different departments of the organization work. It's not just a 30- or 90-day program either. Set the stage for ongoing professional development beyond the initial orientation experience.

In the end, don't neglect the closure of the formal orientation period, which provides a sense of accomplishment and a rite of passage. Celebrate a successful onboarding with the preceptor and fellow staff members. Our team bought silver-colored trays and plastic champagne glasses from a discount store so we could share a toast (with ginger ale, of course). We even cut a piece of tube gauze stretched between the preceptor and new hire to represent cutting the umbilical cord. The gesture was symbolic, meaningful, and the cost was minuscule.

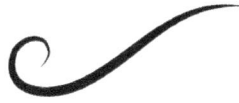

Performance Reviews

I planned annual vacations in the Outer Banks of North Carolina and would head down I-664 every autumn soon after completing the last evaluation. In some magical way, tension and pressures vanish as weary travelers soak in the majestic beauty and traverse the captivating Wright Memorial Bridge into Kitty Hawk. Anyone who has ever been to the region will agree simply crossing over the inlet known by locals as "the sound" is a cathartic experience. I needed this retreat to the shores of the Atlantic after the whirlwind of meetings and the stress of deadlines characteristic of the annual review process.

Although some managers with merely a few employees effortlessly completed this task, I had roughly 60 staff members and occasionally more direct reports. Given the sheer number of evaluations, it would have been easier to have an indolent "place a checkmark in the box" mentality, but then evaluations would have been a waste of everyone's time.

Instead of taking the easy road, I chose to use the annual evaluation period to motivate workers, make a case for pay increases, ask *stay* questions to get views on what employees like about their work and what could be improved. Include positive feedback during the annual review process. After all, a person who has no way of knowing they are doing a good job will become frustrated. Imagine playing a hockey game and not knowing the score or being a stockbroker and not knowing if the value went up or down after you traded.

Evaluations are also prime times for discussing developmental opportunities. Such was the case one year when I was on the receiving end of a performance evaluation from a boss named Amy.

Amy tailored the performance appraisals to match my personality and managerial position. The sessions were more consultative than traditional evaluations and were always stellar—until one year. On this occasion, Amy's assessment of my performance was middle-of-the-road at best. Yet, I had a perfect attendance record, always reported on time, and fulfilled my duties. Fortunately, I was assertive enough to ask why I didn't receive higher ratings, such as *exceeds expectations* when working many long and hard hours.

At this juncture, it's helpful to know some background about a form of philosophy I designated "Amyism." Amyism champions the advice Jedi Master Yoda asserted in *The Empire Strikes Back.* "Do or Do Not. There is no try." In other words, deliver on commitments.

Sometimes it's not enough to do our best. Sometimes it's not acceptable to say I tried. You must deliver. We don't get paid for trying. People generally pay us for delivering products or services. Effort is not rewarded. Outcomes, deliverables, quality, and performance matter. Simply, results override busyness.

When I reflect upon this evaluation, I'm reminded of a hamster on a wheel who is very busy but not getting anywhere. As Amy explained, it's not about the number of hours I put in, but about the difference I was making. Effort is only part of the process of getting there.

In short, a lot of effort that doesn't lead to outcomes will not be rewarded. Don't confuse deliverable quantity with quality. Professionals have a bias for results. The wonderful irony is I learned to deliver on commitments and still have down time because the emphasis was on results, not busyness. Now, that's the power of an effective evaluation.

Performance Appraisals Do's and Don'ts

We must exercise critical thinking skills to see through to the heart of something accurately, such as performance in this case. Critical thinking means we conduct an objective analysis to form a judgment and thwart hasty generalizations, such as the halo and horn biases. Just because an employee excels in one area does not mean they do in every domain. Likewise, simply because someone has one weakness does not mean the overall rating should be low.

Another common bias to avoid is the recency effect. Recency occurs when an appraiser gives more weight to current occurrences and discounts earlier performance. There is a tendency for some people to focus on what's happened lately when evaluating or judging someone. Some managers tend to weigh what the employee has done in the last weeks or months rather than looking at the entire evaluation period. Remember, too, recent behavior can be positive or negative, so managers with a recency bias may be evaluating overly positive or negative, depending on what's most proximate.

Three other mistakes come to mind, especially when using rankings or numeric scales for evaluations.

Strictness: The supervisor will not give high ratings. For example, on a scale from one to five, the supervisor avoids ratings of five because the highest score suggests perfection. This is a fallacy because evaluations typically refer to behaviors occurring 80% of the time, not all of the time.

Central Tendency: All employees are rated in a narrow mid-range regardless of performance.

Leniency: Appraisers don't want to give anyone a low score. Be especially careful to avoid inflating the assessment of an employee. You may need documentation of performance later, and it must be factual. If you terminate an employee, they usually should not have a stellar evaluation in their personnel file.

To help avoid these pitfalls, ask employees to bring supporting documentation, such as portfolios with achievements, certifications, awards, and thank-you notes to incorporate into the review. Additionally, conversations should occur throughout the year as an ongoing, continuous process. There should never be any big surprises during an evaluation.

Lastly, remember to include goal setting for the subsequent assessment, focusing on performance in support of strategic goals. Strategically focused objectives help create a clear line of sight from individual efforts to the organization's success. Your job as a leader is to help employees connect the dots and understand how what they do every day helps the organization move forward and accomplish the larger overarching goals.

You've probably written SMART goals, but there is a SMARTER method to ensure employees know what is expected of them at work every day.

Specific: Focus the goal on a narrowly defined activity rather than a generalization. Be as specific as possible about the result you want to accomplish.

Measurable: The desired outcome is capable of objective measurement to help you hold people (or yourself) accountable. What gets measured gets done! Note even intangibles can be measured objectively once a measurement system is established. Provide the baseline data, which is a step often missed. Explain where we are now in relation to the desired future.

Attainable and Agreed: The goal should require effort and be achievable given the right tools and support. Set the bar at the right level. People want stretching but realistic goals. Of equal importance, targets are more likely to be attained when both the manager and individual agree on desired results. There will be no ownership and individuals can even become resistant when managers force objectives upon them.

Relevant: The goal must be meaningful and aligned with the overarching goals of the organization. Is the goal a priority?

Timebound: Subject the goal to evaluation within a reasonable and defined time frame. Immediacy is important so people will begin to work on the goal. There must be a specific amount of time or a realistic deadline for accomplishing the results. If necessary, break down the goals into short-term and long-term segments and establish dates for deliverables.

Evaluated: Assess the goal at the designated time or interval, often continuously in the form of progress reports or pulse checks. Take stock of everything you've accomplished and celebrate success.

Revised: Goals are amended to reflect what has been learned during the evaluation. Repeat the objective-setting process to ensure the activities chosen are still relevant and the results are attainable.

This final step will drive performance to even higher levels because you learned by following this process and became SMARTER!

Reflection

1. A new manager approaches you with a question about the phenomenon of recency bias. There is an employee who shows significant recent improvement and appears to be on the road to success. Should this employee still be penalized by what happened ten months ago? Should the evaluation still reflect the entire time period or only what is proximate?

2. Develop a minimum of three *stay* questions to provide insight into what is going right. For example, "What are you learning here?" or "On your commute to work, what things do you look forward to?"

3. Develop at least three *stay* questions to give insight on opportunities for improvement. For example, "What can I do to make your experience at work better for you?" or "When was the last time you thought about leaving and what prompted it?"

4. Ask your HR representative to provide statistical data on the most recent appraisals that you completed on your subordinates. Evaluate the information with consideration to strictness, leniency, and central tendency.

5. Write one SMARTER objective directly related to a personal goal. For example, if your goal is related to fitness, write something more than "I want to prepare for a charitable 3K event scheduled later this year." Instead write, "I will record a minimum of 4,000 steps (approximately 2 miles) on a pedometer daily in time frames not exceeding 45 mins. for the next 8 weeks. After 2 months, I will evaluate my goal and make adjustments as needed."

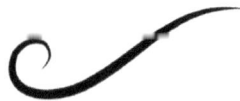

Crucial Conversations

I've talked with low performers who were surprisingly very adept when it came to having difficult conversations. I finally figured out why: they have been practicing since the third grade! As a leader, you must be as experienced in the art of crucial conversations as they are. You cannot sidestep difficult discussions when there are conflicting opinions and emotions are running high. It's far better to face and deal with situations directly than to avoid or ignore them. It's a competency we must learn, practice, and refine. Let's look at some lessons from my own experience.

First, plan the crucial conversations at the right time, in the right place, with the right words, and with the right approach. Don't let things fester before taking action. Schedule a timely discussion after you have had time to calm down and think about what you will say. I sometimes need to take a time-out before responding to a personal triggering event. Keep the conversations as confidential as possible and in a private space. Choose words with the intent of raising others up, not tearing them down. Before meeting with the individual, determine the best approach, such as the method described below.

Your Turn, My Turn

A mentor once told me, "Always assume good intentions." A good premise is people typically come to work wanting to do a good job. Therefore, when an employee's performance is deficient, consider whether or not proper instructions were given, if the person had adequate training, or if there is some personal issue of which you are unaware.

In other words, approach difficult discussions from a curiosity mindset rather than leading with a negative mindset, conclusions, and emotions. It took time for me to learn the importance of deferring judgment. More often than not, things did not turn out the way I expected when I had preconceived opinions.

Consequently, I changed my approach after learning the "Your Turn, My Turn" method. It's simple and works because people don't become defensive. The technique was exactly what I needed to remedy the habit of jumping to conclusions.

You begin by using communication builders like, "One of the reasons we are meeting is because I want you to be successful in your role, and I have something I would like to share because it may help make you become more effective." Then, in the next 30 seconds or so, tell the person what you want to discuss. Remain constructive, specific, and focused on verifiable facts to capture the situation and describe behavior. Then, stop right there and ask them to explain. "What do you know about this?" They get the first turn. Don't interrupt except to paraphrase for understanding.

Next, ask to explain your point of view. It's important to realize we don't need to go too far into the conversation from our perspective. Again, you have communicated your desire for the person to be successful on the job, so identifying the specific behaviors impeding their success and the impact of those actions will help you move the discussion forward and develop a plan of action. You need to create a two-way conversation. One of the benefits of this method is parties work together to identify problems and find solutions. You both have a shared investment in the outcomes.

As a cautionary note, avoid two common blunders. First, don't play games like "sandwiching," which puts a brief reference to the actual problem between two complementary phrases or charades where you hope the other person will guess the problem from hints.

Secondly, never pass the buck. For example, don't say, "I don't really want to suspend you, but I've been ordered by HR and my boss to take disciplinary action. I don't have a choice." Making someone else responsible for a problem you should deal with only serves to undermine your authority.

After the discussion, document the conversation's crucial points, any relevant policies, and actions taken, such as a performance improvement plan. Ensure you and the other person agree on the next steps and how you will work together to meet your respective goals and attain positive outcomes within a specified timeframe.

Reflection

1. Describing behavior can be difficult. Read the list below and circle phrases describing behavior.

> He was rude.
> She was preoccupied.
> He seemed bored with the presentation.
> She was arrogant.
> He appeared very aggressive.

If you didn't circle any, then you're on track. The above list includes adjectives describing the observer's interpretation or impression—not specific actions.

2. Rewrite each phrase with a focus on action(s). For example, "Jim, during the staff meeting on Tuesday afternoon, I noticed you tapped your pencil loudly, interrupted other people, and rolled your eyes while Sarah was speaking" (*rude*). Remember to communicate the impact of the person's behavior on you, your team, and the organization. "These actions diminish the team's productivity and cohesiveness."

I'll stop right here. It's your turn.

Without a doubt, Human Resources is a broad and complex topic. Fortunately, we are not on an island. Remember, when in doubt, utilize the expertise and experience of HR practitioners.

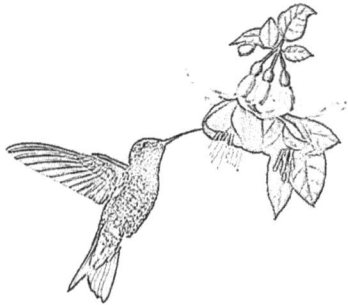

Part Three

Chapter Seven:
Clinical Notes and Stretcher-Side Lessons

You treat a disease, you win, you lose. You treat a person, I guar-antee you, you'll win, no matter what the outcome.

- Patch Adams (Shadyac, 1998, 1:43)

Lesson One: Sandbox 101

Be Safe and Be Kind

Forty years ago, I learned the most important lesson of my entire career: *Primum non nocere*. We can trace the origin of this maxim back hundreds of years. First, do no harm, or more simply, be safe.

Healthcare is a high-risk industry with devastating consequences when mistakes, such as medication errors, are made. There are countless tragic stories of patients killed and injured by experienced, caring professionals—good people—who went to work one day and made a deadly error. We all have close calls and make errors of varying severity, regardless of our knowledge. No one is immune from making mistakes.

The key to dealing effectively with near misses and slips is to embrace them, learn from them, and share lessons to build competence, not only in your department but throughout the organization. It is also incumbent to not be judgmental. Sometimes the mistake is not as painstaking as how your peers make you feel after the mistake. We should learn from everyone's mistakes. After all, "No one is always right, and everyone is sometimes wrong" (Richard Paul Evans, 2020, p.177).

As a leader, you are ultimately responsible for making sure the organization is safe. This essential role is accomplished by establishing clear expectations for safe behaviors and managing accountability to ensure they are met. Accountability is NOT about punishing people but rather about counting on them to take responsibility for their work. Accountability also involves answering to results—good and bad—while learning and growing when things don't entirely go as expected.

Supervisors, managers, and other overseers show the way with straightforward, easy-to-follow rules and directions. There's a fine line between micromanagement and thorough oversight. Nevertheless, you can stay in your administrative lane while steering others in the right direction and lowering risks. Risk reduction strategies include clearly defining critical rules, communicating consequences of violations, and providing tools (procedures and processes, equipment, job aids, and guardrails) to support a safe practice environment.

Here's one example of a clearly defined rule. Do not distract nurses in the process of removing drugs from the medication dispensing machine. Naturally, new practices are most effective when they are "sticky," meaning changes are readily retained and adopted. One ED manager used the ultimate easy solution to make this rule stick. She purchased brightly colored duct tape to partition a four-by-four "Do Not Disturb" zone around the MedStation. No interruptions were permitted when a nurse occupied the square except in rare and emergent situations. This approach worked well (even though employees jumped inside the box whenever the manager walked by). The teasing and good humor functioned as an extra behavioral anchor. The rule was sticking! Sometimes simple solutions work best.

Red Rules

Many high-risk industries and organizations have adopted red rules—rules which cannot be broken. These rules are limited to processes that, if not followed, may result in severe harm or death to customers and workers. If you're not in the healthcare profession, there are also red rules applicable to everyone's life, for example, the use of seatbelts. Suppose a vehicle occupant is not buckled up when the auto is placed in drive. Any person in the car (children included) should be comfortable speaking up to tell the person not wearing the seatbelt to buckle up. The vehicle's driver should halt until the seatbelt is fastened and secured. If the individual refuses to comply, then consequences may follow, such as a ticket for the violation or even bodily harm from a crash.

What would happen if an environmental service (EVS) worker spoke up because a nurse and physician omitted a timeout before beginning an invasive procedure? How would your team handle a similar situation? Would everyone immediately halt the process and say, "You are correct," then perform the mandatory timeout to verify patient identity, the procedure, and site? Your answer will reveal telling information about the organizational culture.

Incidentally, this was an actual event. An EVS employee learned about red rules while attending a hospital-wide safety fair. Soon after the training, a nurse and physician arrived to perform a bedside thoracentesis just as the housekeeper finished cleaning the area. The EVS worker expected to hear a "timeout" as she pushed her cart away. She listened as she left but didn't hear anything resembling the timeout explained at the safety training. At this point, it may have been easier to leave and perhaps discuss the incident with a supervisor at a later time or ignore it altogether. Instead, the EVS worker courageously spoke up and asked, "Is this one of those operations where everybody is supposed to stop and do a checklist first?" What happened next? The team members, including the physician, were receptive and even thanked her for the gentle nudge, then conducted the timeout. The story of the EVS Hero spread like wildfire.

Highlighting stories like this will make rules stick. Without a doubt, timeouts are deep-rooted in this organization's culture. Do you have a story to share?

Be Kind

After safety, the next priority is simply being kind—do unto others the way you would your friends and family. Notably, this tenet also applies to your co-workers. When faced with a difficult decision, we should consider how we would treat loved ones. Following this rule can sometimes be difficult, especially when others have habits or behaviors we dislike. Regardless, listen to your patients and show them you care. We are here to treat and care, not to judge.

Indeed, it is a conundrum that the patient is the least utilized resource in healthcare, yet the essence for our existence. There is value in sharing positive and negative excerpts from patient satisfaction surveys with all team members. All we need to do is connect the dots to see the link between perceptions of compassionate care and opinions about competence levels.

Patient satisfaction does influence perceptions of the quality of care delivered (Brosinski & Riddell, 2020). This correlation is evident even when commendatory, "glowing" patient satisfaction surveys are not indicative of what professionals consider quality patient care. No one wants nurses at the bedside who are unkind, abrasive, or insensitive, regardless of their skill level. Have you ever seen a thank-you note for the way a nurse expertly titrated an intravenous medication drip? As stated before, no one cares how much you know until they know how much you care. It's about how you made the patient feel—the human connection. Be kind.

The sequential order and relationship between safety, customer service, and quality of care can be summarized with the mantra:

Be safe (do no harm),

Be kind,

Make the patient better if you can (do good),

In that order,

And you will win, every time.

Reflection

1. What are the red rules in your workplace?

2. When a red rule is not being followed, are all your employees, regardless of position, empowered to speak up and "stop the line?"

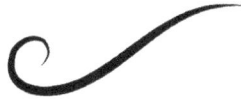

Lesson Two: The Win Principle

Now, tune your radio dial to WIIFM (*What's in it for me?*) as we break for a brief commercial announcement.

Broadcaster: "Listeners, do you want to gain a competitive edge? Generate more revenue? Grow to become the leader in your industry? If so, adopt a patient-centric strategy because *what is best for the customer is also best for you.* Profits will follow when caregivers are attentive to patients' preferences, needs, and values. The subsequent increase in the operating margin will generate a means to extend your mission further, resulting in growth! For the best results, apply the WIN Principle each day by asking:

What's Important Now?

The answer will always be the patient.

In the world of finance, a thought-provoking but obsolete adage is *volume hides all sins.* We sometimes gloss over expenses and labor productivity numbers that are a little out of line when patient volume is high. The operational costs get buried in the overall size of the volume. Yet, the healthcare industry moved away from a volume-based system to a value-based system. Hospitals and practitioners are now paid based on patient health outcomes. Today, the financial management approach you take when the volume is high should be the same as when the volume is down. Always be attentive to value, efficiency, patient satisfaction percentiles, and positive outcome measures. Remember:

Profits = Operating Margin and Mission
It's a win/win!

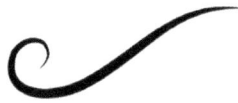

Lesson Three: Document, Document, Document

Good documentation promotes patient safety and quality of care. The following tips do not constitute legal advice; however, the recommendations may improve the ability of legal counsel to provide an affirmative defense if one is required. Unfortunately, these are litigious times.

Monitors are machines. *You* are a critical thinker. Do not select auto populate and pull invalid data, such as vital signs, into the medical record. For example:

Time 2015: Pulse 84, Respirations 16, B/P 124/72, Pulse Oximetry 20% on room air.

Years from now, you may have to explain away the erroneous pulse oximeter reading entered into the medical record (the patient's hand was cold, the patient was moving her hand, or the probe was off). Moreover, don't merely document vital signs but also report and act upon any abnormal findings. Document your actions, including M.D. notification, such as "MD (name) acknowledged receipt of information," and any orders received.

Before you write *vital signs are stable,* you must first ask, "Are the vital signs normal?" The dead are always stable.

Assessments: Base focused reassessments on the chief problem. For example, are the presenting symptoms still there? "Family at bedside" is not a reassessment! Also, avoid the abbreviation WNL for within normal limits. It also means "We Never Looked!"

Be attentive to details, such as laterality. Speak up when a discrepancy occurs to prevent wrong-side and wrong-site procedures, such as x-rays and surgeries.

Be careful documenting "unwilling." Perhaps the patient was actually "unable."

Providing discharge instructions is an excellent use of your time. Include written instructions in the patient's preferred language and in an appropriate font style and size. Emphasize critical information. Discharge instructions should be achievable, patient-specific, and concise. No one will read pages and pages of standardized, generic computer-generated instructions, yet we often provide the equivalent of a medical textbook.

Additionally, avoid giving ranges, such as "follow-up in one to two weeks" and vague terms, such as "push fluids." Provide a teach-back which is a confirmation method to validate the patient understands what is being explained. Include significant others when giving instructions, when possible.

Confirm an *accurate* contact number in case a call back is required. Explain a follow-up notification may be necessary in the event of a discrepancy or to discuss pending results, such as positive cultures.

Avoid superfluous, disparaging remarks in the medical record. For example, "Frequent flyer well known to the ED presents with drug-seeking behavior."

Never point fingers, blame others, document fault, or "argue" in the medical record. An example of this is, "The patient fell off the stretcher because the technician left the rail down after drawing labs."

Lastly, always avoid unapproved abbreviations and spelling errors, such as qd. When in doubt, write it out.

Sometimes you win . . .
and sometimes you learn
(The Hard Way).

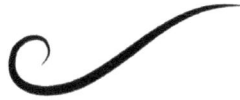

Lesson Four: The Emergency Department is the Great Equalizer

Nothing good ever happens in an ED waiting room, with one exception: Triage areas are "Great Equalizers." You may be beautiful, rich, and famous in life, but the ED levels the playing field. Upon arrival to the ED, the only thing that matters is the severity of one's illness or injury.

Many ED nurses have received a notification to expect the arrival of a board member, famous actor, staff physician or nurse, local news celebrity, or some other influential person and even family members of the above. The unspoken expectation is to see them more quickly, be more attentive, and assign the patient to the most experienced providers. This has the potential to substantially disrupt the delivery of care to other patients. It also creates cynicism among staff. There should be zero tolerance for preferential treatment based on anything other than the reason for seeking care. Favoritism is ethically inappropriate and may even violate privacy laws.

So, the next time you are sitting in an ED waiting room, remember this lesson. You're one of the lucky ones. An emergency department is somewhere you don't want to be a very important person (VIP)—the number one priority holding the winning ticket. Yes, you may get to go ahead of everyone else, but the only reason is that you may die or suffer permanent disability without immediate care.

Sometimes it is better not to win!

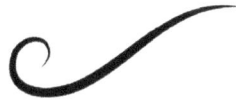

Lesson Five: De-Ass the Chair at Triage and in the Nurses' Station

Triage tools, such as the Emergency Severity Index, help registered nurses discriminate between patients requiring emergent care and those who can wait. Yet, even the best triage tools are not a substitute for rounding in the waiting area, hence this lesson: DE-ASS the Chair.

Get out of the chair to summon patients to the triage area rather than calling names over an intercom while planted behind a barrier. Why is this important? The initial component of the triage process is an "across the room assessment" to evaluate the general appearance and detect obvious alterations to airway, breathing, circulatory status, or neurological condition. At this stage, you are often able to identify patients with potentially life-threatening or debilitating conditions. Another reason for going to where the patients are is to offer assistance, such as a wheelchair for safety.

Additionally, you are making first impressions which will set the stage for the entire emergency department visit. Approach every person seeking care as though they are a close friend or family, treating them with courtesy and respect.

Lastly, there's something in it for you, too—exercise! I have always been perplexed when nurses are assigned to triage because they are on "light duty" or "need a break." Please don't do it!

Triage nurses must be capable of rapidly pivoting to meet the ever-changing demands and workload. Only the fittest and smartest nurses with the strongest interpersonal skills belong at triage. Should I add bravest?

While assigned to triage, make frequent rounds in the waiting area. The patients' perception of quality decreases proportionately to the length of wait time. Begin treatment and testing as soon as possible, such as applying ice packs and elevating injured extremities, removing rings to prevent injury from swelling, obtaining laboratory studies and x-rays, and other modalities based on pre-approved orders. Assess and reassess patients while also keeping them informed while they wait.

One evening the emergency department was bustling when a thin, tall adolescent male arrived and signed in with a chief complaint of difficulty breathing. He did not seem to be in respiratory distress from across the room, although he appeared mildly anxious. There were approximately five people signed in ahead of him. Due to the volume of patients presenting simultaneously, I rounded in the waiting room to prioritize new arrivals. When I reached the young man, he stated he just coughed and then felt a sharp pain in his chest followed by shortness of breath. His breath sounds were markedly diminished on one side when I auscultated his chest. I reached for his wrist and noted a rapid pulse rate. I immediately triaged him to the main treatment area, notified the physician, and requested a stat portable chest x-ray. Early identification of a spontaneous pneumothorax prevented a life-threatening condition. My first thought was, "There but for the grace of God go I." My triage seat never gets too warm.

Purposeful Rounding

Similarly, the default position should be at the bedside (or stretcher-side) in the treatment area, not sitting as inconspicuous as possible behind a computer at the desk.

Downtime in an emergency department is specious (unless you are a computer). A few simple measures, such as rounding, will enhance the patients' experiences, reduce their anxiety, improve the perception of care, and promote safety. Rounding will also reduce call lights which is a smart time management strategy. Caregivers who systematically and proactively perform rounding take control of their time rather than reacting to call bells. What's best for the patient is also best for you.

Tips on Rounding:

Pause at the threshold and take a few calming breaths before knocking to enter a patient's room.

Always use the patient's name and at least one additional identifier, such as the patient's date of birth.

Narrate and describe actions while performing tasks, such as hand hygiene when entering the room. We want patients to remember we washed our hands every time we entered and exited the room.

Momentarily sit and make eye contact (eye to eye and heart to heart). Patients may perceive you spent more time at the bedside and listened more intently if you took a seat.

Invest time in patient education to foster self-care.

Remember the Seven Ps.

Pain assessment: Follow your organizational policy on pain management and recommendations for reassessment.

Positioning: Ask about comfort. Provide a blanket and pillow, as needed.

Periphery: Complete a safety check of the room. Ensure a tidy and clean environment.

Plug in electrical equipment: Check pumps.

Place personal items within reach: Can they reach the call bell and phone? Arrange the overbed table.

Potty: Ask about bathroom needs.

Privacy: Improve the atmosphere by turning down lights, limiting noise, and providing privacy. Ask if they would like their door closed for *privacy*.

Empower frontline staff to implement measures for service recovery as needed. For example, write a policy and establish an account or system with the gift shop so charge nurses or team leaders can purchase flowers, balloons, cards, or stuffed animals for patients. Staff members should not have to come to the director or manager for every menial purchase, such as buying a card when realizing it's a patient's birthday.

What's the difference between ordinary and extraordinary?

Winners know it is the little extra effort and energy that creates a triumph!

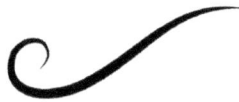

Lesson Six: Use All of Your Senses

(Even the Sixth Sense and Always Common Sense)

If you're an ED nurse, you likely encounter many people whose powers of reasoning and decision-making processes look like this:

That's no sense and nonsense! On the other hand, the best nurses and doctors use common sense every day. They know when we hear hoofbeats, we should first think of horses, not zebras.

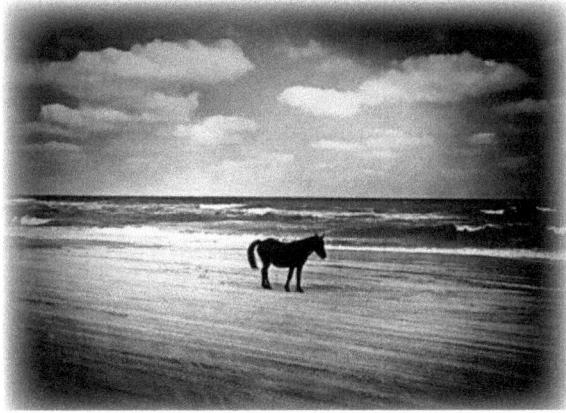

Keep your eyes open for common red flags. For example, an insulin-dependent diabetic presents to the ED with non-specific and non-diagnostic symptoms of cool, clammy skin, a rapid pulse, and altered mental status. What is the most likely cause? A transient ischemic attack? A psychological condition? A rare enzyme deficiency? Those are zebras. Common sense dictates hypoglycemia is the most likely reason for the patient's symptoms.

Use all your senses: sight, hearing, touch, taste, smell—even your sixth sense—with every patient contact. Put your hands on the patient to assess pulses, skin temperature, and moisture. This simple maneuver alone provides an abundance of important information.

The sense of smell to identify odors can be specific to a patient's condition, such as foul odors due to tissue breakdown. Assess body and breath odors, which might indicate alcohol intoxication, poor hygiene, or metabolic acidosis. The senses of smell and taste may even help you to detect harmful chemicals in the air or poisons.

Most seasoned nurses and physicians also develop a sixth sense which triggers a visceral response when something "just doesn't feel right." It's when the hair on the back of your neck stands up, but you can't seem to put your finger on why. Trust the feeling in your gut and dig deeper. Don't be concerned about what others may think if it turns out you're wrong.

One early evening around dinnertime, a seven-year-old male was brought to the ED by his mother following a bicycle fall. There were no visible signs of injury except for minor abrasions, vital signs were age-appropriate, and he had no complaints except related to his wrecked bike. He had a helmet on at the time of the accident. The mother stated she witnessed the bicycle tire hit the curb and saw him fly over the handlebars.

The emergency department was hectic as usual on a Monday. I didn't have any objective data for why I immediately took him to the treatment area ahead of many other "low acuity" patients. Shortly thereafter, the child began to complain of abdominal tenderness beneath his left ribcage and left shoulder pain. The physician diagnosed a ruptured spleen and transferred the child in stable, but guarded, condition to another facility for definitive care. To this day, I don't know why I took him back without delay. A nurse's intuition?

A combination of critical thinking and intuition equals a win every time.

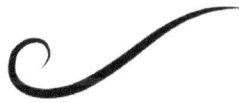

Lesson Seven: Nakedness is Next to Godliness

Mothers often tell their children to "always wear clean underwear in case of an accident!" As if nurses and doctors have never seen dirty underwear. Forget the underwear! Better advice is to teach patients to empty their bladders before getting into cars.

A person's bladder can rupture if it is full, especially when wearing a low-fitting seatbelt at the time of a crash. Besides, in many emergencies such as traumas, we cut clothes off anyway. It is the "Naked Truth."

Healthcare providers should also routinely remove clothing to assess pediatric patients. It's an opportunity to detect bruising—a common sign of physical abuse—and other hidden injuries that would go unnoticed otherwise.

For obvious reasons, we must remove clothing for specific studies, such as bras which obscure images on chest x-rays. Clothing often contains hidden metal such as zippers (even metallic threads) which can be hazardous in a magnetic resonance imaging (MRI) scan.

The following two incidents epitomize the rationale for naked-ness. The accounts reflect the author's present recollections of experiences over decades. Some characteristics have been altered, and some incidents have been condensed. Names, places, and time periods are excluded from the events.

Case #1: Personnel at a long-term care facility called 911 to request emergency transport for an elderly female with altered mental status. There are so many causes of altered mental status that medical professionals use an acronym (AEIOU-TIPS) to help in the differential diagnosis. O, for example, stands for overdose.

On evaluation, all of her lab studies were normal. She did not suffer from hypoglycemia and did not appear to have an infection (I), both of which often account for decreased mental status in the elderly. A cat scan of her brain revealed mild atrophy but no acute findings.

Meanwhile, a nurse combed through multiple pages of the hand-written medication administration records received from the nursing home. She discovered fentanyl (Duragesic) transdermal patches, a potent opioid, transcribed as an order for every three days. Based on this information, the ED physician prescribed naloxone (Narcan), an opioid antagonist; however, the patient required repeat doses of the antidote.

Finally, the patient was undressed and reexamined. Multiple medication patches peppered her back. A transdermal patch must be removed when a new one is applied, but caregivers were applying new patches every third day and leaving old ones in place. Nakedness is next to Godliness.

Case # 2: On a busy Friday night, Emergency Medical Services (EMS) transported an intoxicated and unruly 26-year-old male to the ED. The paramedics reported police were on the scene and allowed him to choose jail or the ED. He was sober enough to favor the ED. Perhaps because he only had "two beers" (2 x 2 x 2 x2).

On arrival, staff placed him in the de-escalation or "quiet" room due to aggression and agitation. The monitored seclusion room was free of all fixtures, furniture, trash containers, and any potentially harmful devices. A recessed panel securely housed electrical receptacles, medical gas supplies, and other hardware. The door to the seclusion room had an observation pane made of transparent wire glass of sufficient size for someone outside the entrance to monitor the entire space.

The staff was not able to complete a comprehensive initial assessment due to the patient's violent behavior. For safety, four-point leather restraints were ordered and applied by a team of nurses, technicians, and security personnel. Contrary to the hospital's policy on restraints, the staff did not remove the patient's clothes. Per protocol, all restrained patients must be in paper scrubs. Security did not discover any contraband, such as weapons, during the application of restraints. The charge nurse assigned a psychiatric aide to monitor the patient continuously, and a nurse performed assessment checks every fifteen minutes.

After one of the fifteen-minute checks, the nurse left to assess a new admission. Shortly thereafter, the patient ignited his clothing and bed linens with a cigarette lighter. The technician assigned to observe the patient was momentarily distracted by her mobile device.

A team assigned to investigate the sentinel event reviewed footage from a video camera hidden in the seclusion room. The patient managed to reach into his pocket to remove a disposable lighter. No one ever determined his motive for starting the fire. Nakedness is next to Godliness.

To leave garments on is sometimes a sin,
while taking clothes off can lead to a win.
Amen.

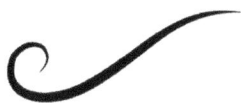

Lesson Eight: Trust No One
(Not Even Yourself and Your Colleagues)

Have you ever been asked this dreaded question from a colleague, *"Hey, remember that patient...?"*

This incomplete sentence alone can precipitate panic and evoke a gut-wrenching feeling.

But wait! There's more.

"You know, the twenty-seven-year-old woman you saw a couple of days ago with chest tightness and mild shortness of breath? She was diagnosed with anxiety and discharged. Well, she returned this morning around six am for worsening dyspnea and chest pain. I ordered a spiral chest CT, but she coded before the scan could be completed and died. I think she may have had a PE (pulmonary embolus). Did you know she just returned from a mission trip abroad?"

Here's the crux: assumptions, biases, or misperceptions (even our own) can befog our thinking and result in errors. A mind is like a parachute; it works best when it is open. Yet, one of the issues with "seasoned" emergency clinicians is much of what we encounter in our daily practice appears obvious. For the most part, it is.

Nonetheless, if I told you there was only one venomous serpent in a bucket with ninety-nine nonpoisonous snakes, would you be willing to place your hand into it? Herein lies the problem with the "narcotizing" effect of obvious—it's only accurate 99% of the time (Weinstock et al., 2006). Maintain an ever-present cognizance of

166

what can go wrong (i.e., worse case scenarios) and a high index of suspicion that things are not always as they first appear.

A resource falling within the category of edutainment (highly educational while entertaining) is *Bouncebacks! Emergency Department Cases: ED Returns*. It's a well-thumbed, dog-eared manual of case scenarios where something went wrong, and there was another chance to get it right. A good rule of thumb is to be hypervigilant when patients "bounce back" to your emergency department.

Over time, most ED personnel naturally develop well-tuned B.S. detectors and rarely placed blind trust in anyone. The ED is an excellent classroom for learning to spot deception! People are unreliable narrators and often tell half-truths or outright lie about how much they drink (always multiply the answer by two), smoking habits, recreational drug use, age, sexual histories, abortions, and surgeries. Some patients may answer yes to every question asked. We don't want perfect; we just want honest! I've seen patients answering yes when questioned about feeling nauseous, only pausing to load a handful of chips into their mouths.

Even with our colleagues, it's best to rely on facts and verify with direct observation. The following occurrence is a case in point. One morning shortly after the night crew went home, a nurse began assessments and found an elderly patient with a hip deformity on the floor in a puddle of watery stool. The intravenous bag was dry, and the foley catheter bag was full with tubing tangled in the rail.

The nurses had conducted the entire shift report while sitting at the nurses' station. Again, "de-ass" the chair. Bedside handoffs drive accountability for completing tasks and care, keep patients better informed, provide assurance the patient's condition is consistent with the report, and strengthen teamwork.

I couldn't help but ask, "Why did you accept the assignment without rounding?" This question became my rote response when nurses and technicians complained rooms were left unclean, bedpans and urinals unemptied, and rooms unstocked. It didn't take long for the NBC (nagging, bitching, and complaining) program series to end.

Finally, think twice when co-workers and other intelligent people disagree with you. Encourage a curiosity mindset. Sometimes we need to let go of our initial impressions and be attentive to others' informed opinions and objective data. It's equally imperative to avoid notions of hierarchy, such as between attending physicians and nurses. It's not only acceptable for nurses to probe questionable physician orders and verbalize concerns; it's a professional duty.

What if a nurse had questioned the discharge order for the twenty-seven-year-old female with chest tightness and mild shortness of breath? What if she had inquired about risk factors for deep vein thrombosis and pulmonary embolism, such as prolonged inactivity during travel? What if all nurses felt empowered to speak up? What if . . . ? Even if you graduated from nursing school only yesterday, you are already capable of offering an opinion to save a life.

Want to be trusted? Win it.

Reflection

Handoffs can be added as a topic for daily team huddles. It can be fun, such as asking everyone to complete this sentence:

Have you ever walked into a room after completing a shift report *without* bedside rounds and . . .

- thought to yourself, "*I don't know who she gave her report on! This woman is very sick!*"
- found the IV bag empty and the Foley bag overflowing?
- the patient asked with a quiver in her voice, "Who are you? You're not my nurse!"
- discovered an empty stretcher with a positive gown sign?
- found a piece of equipment you didn't know how to operate?

Your Turn: Add two examples to complete the sentence.

Have you ever walked into a room after completing a shift report *without* bedside rounds and . . .

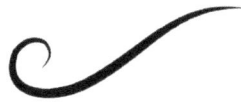

Lesson Nine: Be Attentive to Transitions in Care

In addition to handoffs at shift change, *any* transfer of care from one area or caregiver to another is a critical time interval with the most significant risk for patient harm. These transitions of patient care, especially interdepartmental handoffs, are fraught with dangers due to omissions, fragmented care, and loss of vital information.

Accountability issues related to ambiguous role responsibility may also occur at the point of handoff. For example, what procedure do you follow if a laboratory technician notifies the emergency department of a critical or "panic" lab result, such as a dangerously low potassium level, after moving the patient to an inpatient unit? A faulty assumption is the inpatient nurse will follow up on ED laboratory or radiology test results or even be aware of abnormal findings. This could result in a deadly delay in treatment.

What can you do to ensure a safe passage? One technique is incorporating recommendations and providing anticipatory guidance during handoffs, such as discussing what is most worrisome or what could go wrong. For example, in a patient admitted for diabetic ketoacidosis, the ED nurse may advise a novice RN to monitor the serum potassium as the glucose levels normalize. Don't be afraid to make recommendations or state, "I suggest you . . ." (what needs to be followed up on or monitored). Handoffs also frequently involve the concomitant transfer of special equipment and appliances that may require instruction.

Also, consider innovative solutions to handoff processes, such as admission procedures from the emergency department to inpatient units. What if I told you there are unconventional methods to improve interdepartmental collaboration, promote patient/family-centered care and satisfaction, reduce adverse events, affirm admission to the appropriate level of care, enhance continuity of care, and positively affect revenue? Would you try one?

I'm not suggesting we streamline operations with a fleet of drones hovering in our halls to locate nurses and parachute reports to them (not yet).

(Disclaimer: I would not call the following example a best practice since it requires additional research to determine efficacy. Additionally, the reference to the MEWS system is for illustrative purposes only, and similar instruments are available that may be equally or more efficacious.)

Why not have a designated admission/transport RN come to the ED to perform a bedside handoff? This process has the potential to succeed, but only if it is nurse-driven from the bedside and not by leaders sitting around a table in the boardroom. A performance improvement specialist and others can support team members and perform administrative tasks, such as process flow mapping.

Here is a 30,000-foot view and anecdotal account of how the process may work once the patient is ready for transfer out of the ED to another department:

1. ED RN transmits a standardized report to the receiving unit (use technology to alert receiving nurse and admission/transport nurse the document is available).

2. The receiving RN and designated admission/transport RN review the report. The admission/transport nurse gathers any needed equipment, then goes to the ED (within a designated time frame) to complete a bedside handoff.

3. The handoff includes introductions to the patient and significant others, independent pump checks, safety checks, and addressing any questions or concerns *before* transfer. For example, can we discontinue the Foley catheter? Also, calculate a baseline Modified Early Warning System (MEWS) score. The MEWS score is a simple physiological evaluation tool designed to identify patients with declining conditions. MEWS scoring is based on the principle that early warning signs of clinical instability often precede most adverse events, such as cardiac arrest and death. Patients with elevated MEWS scores may require closer observation, such as in an intensive care setting. Before leaving the ED, the admission/transfer RN may request a higher level of care based on institutional protocols for elevated MEWS scores.

4. Confirm disposition of valuables and home medications. Complete the medication reconciliation before medications are sent home.

5. Remember to manage one another up! Managing up means putting another team member in a positive light in the eyes of a patient. Here is an example: "Hello, Mrs. Justice. Michelle will be your nurse this evening. In fact, I just shared with Michelle the important information about your condition and plan of care. Michelle is a certified emergency nurse who I've known for many years. I always hear nice compliments about her from our patients. She will give you excellent care."

6. If the patient is ready for transport, the admission/transport RN accompanies the patient during transfer with the assistance of ancillary staff. Upon arrival, the admission/transport RN may also assist the inpatient nurse with the admission database and other tasks if another patient is not waiting for transfer.

It didn't take long for nurses to recognize the many benefits of a transport/admission RN position and bedside handoff. In many cases, the admission/transfer RN suggested a higher level of care (such as ICU instead of Telemetry), and the hospitalist modified orders before transfer.

Gone were the days of receiving newly admitted patients on a medical unit with elevated MEWS scores, uncontrolled pain, empty IV bags, infiltrated intravenous lines, with empty stomachs and full bladders. There was a decrease in calls to the nursing supervisor to arrange an urgent transfer to a higher level of care. Likewise, gone were the days of ED nurses waiting for the receiving nurse to finally come into the room to accept a patient, searching for intravenous pumps to exchange, then finally arriving back in the ED and finding a new patient waiting in their assigned cubicle. These depictions of the antiquated admission process remind me of the lyrics to a 1968 song by Mary Hopkin, "Those were the days my friend. We thought they'd never end!"

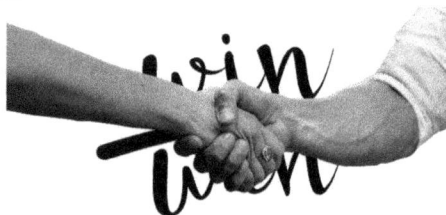

Reflection

As a scholar-practitioner, look to the Emergency Nurses Association (ENA), American Association of Critical Care Nurses (AACN), or other professional organizations for research opportunities on clinical problems encountered in your practice. Remember creativity flourishes in the absence of resources I suppose this means there's never been a better time to begin a new project than now.

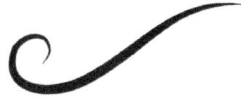

Lesson Ten: Mentor the Next Generation

(If You Ever Want to Retire)

As professionals, it's our duty to "pay it forward." In addition to contributing to the nursing profession through research, mentoring is an opportunity to leave behind a legacy.

Throughout my career, I have been fortunate to learn from many great mentors. I am eternally grateful for their willingness to teach and engage with my desire to learn. I've also discovered unexpected gifts, such as personal resilience, after experiences with a few unkind, unjust, exclusionary, hierarchical, and uncompromising adversaries. The names of these malicious people are . . . no, I don't want to be sued. I'll wait until the depraved are in the grave (I still have a sense of humor).

All wit aside, there will always be a foe lurking in the shadows waiting to ambush. Never run away. Stand and hold your ground. It's analogous to how to keep the situation from escalating when encountering a grizzly bear. If the bear takes notice of you, stay calm, make yourself appear as large as possible, and face the creature directly (National Park Service U.S. Department of the Interior, 2018). Perhaps the bear will recognize you as a human, not prey. Of course, it's best to take steps to avoid an encounter in the first place.

It is also desirable to have a mentor for protection and guidance in the initiation phase of your career. For the old-timers, think of attributes of mentors who had a profound effect on your career and personal life. Some mentors impacted my career development through coaching, promoting competence, and providing career advancement opportunities. Other mentors were more supportive in the psychosocial dimension by counseling, displaying acceptance, role modeling, and friendship. Even now I sometimes think, "What would (mentor's name) do?"

Today you can have a mentoring relationship in the same department or even on the other side of the world. Consider formalized mentoring opportunities, such as the Emergency Nurses Association's Mentoring Program. Find and groom a protégé who will eventually be able to perform your job (only if you ever want to retire). Finally, remember to always surround yourself with good people, and let the others go.

In the end, good people win, and you win with good people.

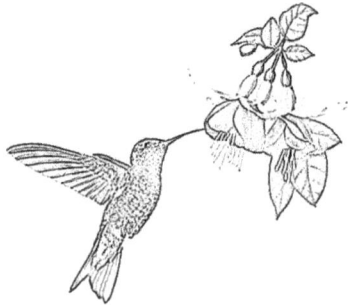

Epilogue

When the door of opportunity closes, another opens; but often we look so long at the closed door we do not see the one which has been opened for us.

– Helen Keller (Koegel, 2007, p. 44)

The challenge now is to determine where you want to start concentrating your efforts in developing your leadership style. What are your vulnerabilities? What can you do to renew yourself? There is a dynamic tension in the gap between where we are today and where we want to be. We never stop growing. We must be committed to lifelong learning, take personal time for quiet incubation of ideas, and practice servitude. This requires a significant and continuous commitment.

Continue reading, networking, and practicing your leadership skills every day. You may even want to begin planning your exit strategy. What do you want people to say about you when you leave your current role? What legacy do you want to leave behind? Don't wait until a deathbed moment to see the differences between how you want to live and how you are living.

If you are already highly successful, don't be paralyzed by past success. Sometimes a successful past blocks our ability to foresee and anticipate what is in the future. Don't take success for granted or become too attached to practices and structures which worked in the past. Similarly, don't stumble and fall over something behind you. We always have to keep pushing forward.

The following may provide a helpful roadmap as you continue your journey:

Things I want to keep doing

Things I want to start doing

Things I want to stop doing (and for which my coworkers and employees will be grateful for the change!)

Finally, go back and review the list of characteristics of leaders outlined in chapter three. Organizations need great leaders who are competent and possess ethics, integrity, and courage. Be one of them.

The Hummingbird

An author's best work comes, not only from the mind, but from the heart and soul. I've saved the best for last. My fourteen-year-old Alaskan Malamute, Johnny, passed away as I was writing this book. My husband, Paul, and I were heartbroken. I began reading a book titled *Signs from Pets in the Afterlife* shortly after our loss. There could not be a better conclusion to a book titled *Leadership in Retrospect* than this passage.

Dear Reader,

Chris and I leave you with this: *What can hummingbirds teach?*

"Able to fly backwards, they educate and inform us that it is okay to look back into our past and revisit those special memories…. We also discover that regret and feelings of guilt are unwarranted" (Ragan, 2015, p. 89).

Take counsel from the past, but do not be ruled by it.

- Stormy and Chris

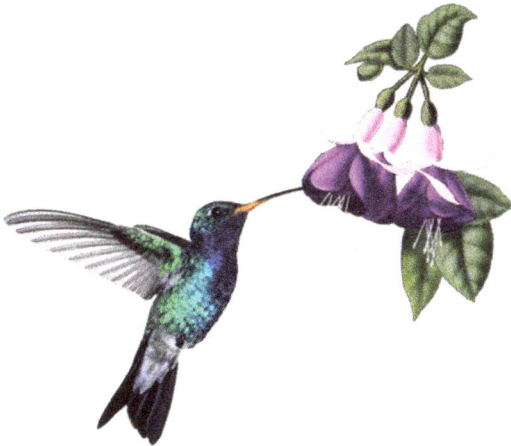

References

A-Z Quotes (n.d.). *Top 25 quotes by Victor E. Frankl (of 215) | A-Z Quotes.* A-Z Quotes.com. Retrieved November 4, 2020, from https://www. azquotes.com/author/5121-Viktor_E_Frankl

Brosinski, C., & Riddell, A. (2020). Incorporating hourly rounding to increase emergency department patient satisfaction: A quality improvement approach. *Journal of Emergency Nursing, 46*(4), 511–517. https://doi.org/10.1016/j.jen.2019.08.004

Cohen, M. H. (2007). *What you accept is what you teach: Setting standards for employee accountability.* Creative Health Care Management.

Copeland, C. L. (2014). *Really important stuff my dog has taught me.* Workman Publishing Co.

Coursen, S. (2021). *The safety trap: A security expert's secrets for staying safe in a dangerous world.* St. Martin's Press.

Covey, S. R. (1989). *The 7 habits of highly effective people: Powerful lessons in personal change.* Fireside Press.

Daft, R. L. (2016). *Organization theory & design* (12th ed.). Cengage Learning.

de Vries, M. K. (2011). *The hedgehog effect: Executive coaching and the secrets of building high performance teams.* Jossey-Bass.

Dominis, M. (2021). Innovation & invention. *ENA Connection, 45*(3), 8–10.

Emerald, D. (2016). *The power of TED: The empowerment dynamic.* Polaris Publishing.

Evans, R. P. (2020). *The Noel letters.* Simon & Schuster.

Fauteux, N. (2021). COVID-19: Impact on nurses and nursing. *AJN, American Journal of Nursing, 121*(5), 19–21. https://doi. org/10.1097/01.naj.0000751076.87046.19

Goldin, K. (2018, October 1). *Great leaders take people where they may not want to go.* Forbes. https://www.forbes.com/sites/kara-goldin/2018/10/01/great-leaders-take-people-where-they-may-not-want-to-go/#483eeea41421

Goleman, D. (2006). *Emotional intelligence.* Bantam Books.

Goodreads (2021). Frank Outlaw > quotes. https://www.goodreads. com/author/quotes/13466663.Frank_Outlaw

Grossman, D., & Christensen, L. W. (2004). *On combat: The psychology and physiology of deadly conflict in war and in peace.* Research Publications.

HIPAA Journal. (2021, January 15). *What are the penalties for HIPAA violations?* HIPAA Journal. https://www.hipaajournal.com/ what-are-the-penalties-for-hipaa-violations-7096/

Jackson, H. (2020). Organizations and organizational design [Lecture notes on mastering organizational effectiveness]. College of Professional Studies, Villanova University. Retrieved from June 30, 2020.

Handbook of wisdom for those in transition. (2008). http://allabout-wichita.com

Koegel, T. J. (2007). *The exceptional presenter: A proven formula to OPEN UP! and own the room.* Greenleaf Book Group Press.

Marquis, B. L., & Carol Jorgensen Huston. (2000). *Leadership roles and management functions in nursing: Theory and application* (3rd ed.). Lippincott Williams & Wilkins.

Merriam-Webster. (1991). *Webster's ninth new collegiate dictionary.*

National Park Service U.S. Department of the Interior. (2018, April 13). *Staying safe around bears.* National Park Service. https://www.nps. gov/subjects/bears/safety.htm#Encounters

O'Toole, G. (2017, February 23). *Good judgment depends mostly on experience and experience usually comes from poor judgment – quote investigator.* Quoteinvestigator.com. https://quoteinvestigator. com/2017/02/23/judgment/

Pink, D. H. (2009). *Drive: The surprising truth about what motivates us.* Riverhead Books.

Pollack, J., & Matous, P. M. (2019, December). *Social network analysis: What it is and why it matters.* www.intheblack.com. https://www.intheblack. com/articles/2019/12/01/what-is-social-network-analysis

Ragan, L. (2015). *Signs from pets in the afterlife: Identifying messages from pets in heaven.*

Reflections in the WORD. (2010, September 15). *A.S.A.P. - Always say a prayer*. https://reflectionsintheword. org/2010/09/15/a-s-a-p-always-say-a-prayer/

Sandel, Donald (2021, April 21). *Resilience and positivity during challenging times* [Webinar]. BCEN Learn. https://learn.bcen.org

Schumaker, J., Taylor, W., & McGonigle, T. (2019). The emergency, trauma, and transport nursing workforce. *Nursing Management (Springhouse)*, *50*(12), 20–32. https://doi.org/10.1097/01. numa.0000605152.42445.4b

Shadyac, T. (Director). (1998). *Patch Adams* [Film; DVD]. Universal Pictures.

Snozek, C. L. H., Hernandez, J. S., & Traub, S. J. (2019). "Rainbow draws" in the emergency department: Clinical utility and staff perceptions. *The Journal of Applied Laboratory Medicine*, *4*(2), 229–234. https://doi.org/10.1373/jalm.2018.027649

Studer Group. (2010). *The nurse leader handbook: The art and science of nurse leadership*. Fire Starter Publishing.

Taylor, H (n.d.). *20 Inspirational Quotes from Jim Rohn*. www.habitsforwell-being.com. Retrieved December 14, 2020, from https://www.habits-forwellbeing.com/20-inspirational-quotes-from-jim-rohn/

Thomas, M. (2018, March 15). To control your life, control what you pay attention to. *Harvard Business Review*. https://hbr.org/2018/03/ to-control-your-life-control-what-you-pay-attention-to

U.S. Department of Health and Human Services. (2013, July 26). *Summary of the HIPAA privacy rule*. HHS.gov. https://www.hhs.gov/hipaa/ for-professionals/privacy/laws-regulations/index.html

Weinstock, M. B., Henry, G. L., Longstreth, R., Meredith, H., & Anadem Publishing. (2006). *Bouncebacks! Emergency department cases: ED returns*. Anadem Publishing.

Widemark, S. (2009). *Lessons from the geese* - Who is the author and is it scientifically sound? Suewidemark.com. http://suewidemark.com/ lessonsgeese.htm

Wikipedia Contributors. (2019a, October 26). *Big stick ideology*. Wikipedia; Wikimedia Foundation. https://en.wikipedia.org/wiki/ Big_Stick_ideology

Wikipedia Contributors. (2019b, December 23). *Peter principle*. Wikipedia; Wikimedia Foundation. https://en.wikipedia.org/wiki/ Peter_principle

Any Internet references contained in the work are current at publication time, but the authors cannot guarantee that a specific location will continue to be maintained.

Image Credits

Image Credits: All images in this book are either original illustrations by Hakm Bin Ahmad, images owned by Antoinette (Stormy) Weathers or Christopher Card, copyrighted images from stock companies that have been purchased and used with permission, the property of other companies used with permission, or are images obtained from the public domain that do not require specific permission for use. A list of credits for these images includes the following:

Ends of Chapters	Hummingbird Sketch designed by Hakm Bin Ahmad
Dedication	Bright star with wings and praying hands. Purchased from iStockphoto.com. ID: 998428872
Page 12	Rainbow in sky, dark and white clouds, lightnings in stormy sky. Purchased from iStockphoto.com. ID: 469047529
Page 14	Nurse with Angel. Image taken by Antoinette Weathers
Page 17	Businessman. Clip art altered for text. Free download
Page 22	Domains of Success. Original figure designed by Antoinette Weathers
Page 26	Pause/Coffee Cup. Purchased from iStockphoto. com. Credit Santje09. ID: 1133163266
Page 27	Lenses. File uploaded: Lenses. Public domain via Wikimedia Commons. https://commons.wikimedia.org
Page 36	I'm Not Bossy! Pinterest.Yourtango.com
Page 49	Batteries. By TheHolloway Tape – Own work, CC By-SA 4.0 https://commons.wikimedia.org/w/index.php?curid=77872129

About the Author

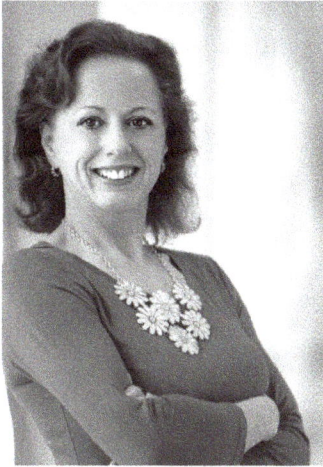

Antoinette Weathers is a self-made professional who has spent a lifetime working in healthcare while continuing her education. She has completed numerous post graduate courses and maintains the highest standards of professional practice. She has maintained her Certification in Emergency Nursing as well membership in the Emergency Nurses Association. With thirty-plus years of experience, she started as a pre-hospital provider and worked in an array of nursing and leadership roles. Now she shares her expertise with readers and various nursing and educational entities as a public speaker and published author. Contact "Stormy" at stormyweathersauthor@gmail.com for bookings, book signings, or engagements.

Christopher Card holds a bachelor's degree in music education, a master's in music education, and a Ph.D. in higher education. As an editor, educator, and music teacher, he has built his career in public, private, and collegiate level schools for two decades. After twenty years in the field, he now consults and teaches privately and writes as well as edits with many projects on the horizon. Contact Chris at cscard@gmail.com for editing or bookings and engagements.

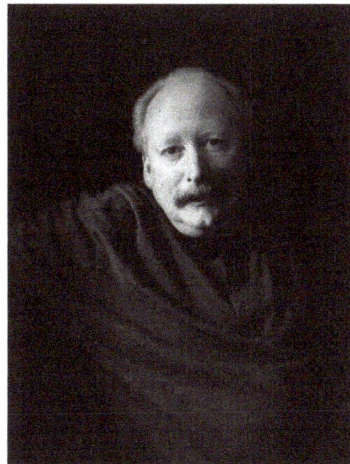

www.ingramcontent.com/pod-product-compliance
Lightning Source LLC
Chambersburg PA
CBHW052113030426
42335CB00025B/2967